REDISCOVERING THE PERSON IN MEDICAL CARE

REDISCOVERING THE PERSON IN MEDICAL CARE

PATIENT · FAMILY
PHYSICIAN · NURSE
CHAPLAIN · PASTOR

JAMES B. NELSON

AUGSBURG PUBLISHING HOUSE
MINNEAPOLIS, MINNESOTA

REDISCOVERING THE PERSON IN MEDICAL CARE

Copyright © 1976 Augsburg Publishing House

Library of Congress Catalog Card No. 76-3858

International Standard Book No. 0-8066-1534-6

Scripture quotations unless otherwise noted are from the Revised Standard Version of the Bible, copyright 1946, 1952, and 1971 by the Division of Christian Education of the National Council of Churches.

MANUFACTURED IN THE UNITED STATES OF AMERICA

Contents

To my brother, Douglas A. Nelson, M.D.

Introduction

The technological aspects of medical care and the ethical issues which they raise have been grist for the mills of Sunday supplements and learned journals alike in recent years. And it is obvious that moral decisions in medicine (or anywhere else) always involve persons and are made by persons. The focus of this volume is less on the medical issues as such than it is on the persons involved. Its focus is more on the *who* question than the *what* question. Surely, the two types of questions, both in theory and in practice, are interrelated. Nevertheless, the main emphasis of the following chapters will fall upon the persons who are making decisions and who are affected by decisions in the medical context. Their ways of perceiving their own identities, their basic beliefs and values, and their ways of looking at the world all inform and shape their actions and responses.

The first essay lifts up some of the underlying belief and value questions which seem to thread their way through the whole gamut of medical-moral issues today. The following two chapters focus on the self-perceptions and identities of two of the many professionals involved in health care—physicians and hospital chaplains. Then we turn to the patient to reflect upon some of his or her needs as a person.

The remaining three chapters attend to particular issues related to persons in medical care. One such matter is human sexuality and sexual health—an area which is only beginning to receive critical attention. The next essay deals with that familiar and difficult scene enacted daily in thousands of hospitals and nursing homes: the interplay of persons as they attempt to make responsible decisions on behalf of a dying patient. The final chapter wrestles with the manner in which our basic values do and will give shape to our patterns of health care; the malpractice insurance problem is its chief illustration.

I have spoken of these chapters as "essays." The dictionary defines that word as follows: "a short literary composition of an analytical or interpretive kind, dealing with its subject usually from a personal point of view or in a limited way." Perhaps that is a reasonably accurate description, and for three reasons.

First, my treatment of these themes is limited. It is limited in the sense of being selective. For example, in addition to the physician and hospital chaplain there are an estimated two hundred different professions and occupations now in the health field. While nurses, administrators, and parish ministers do figure into these pages, there are no separate chapters devoted to them—or to a number of other types of health care persons frequently in relationship with patients and their families. In my selectivity, however, I chose to focus on that medical professional and that religious professional who, in our present situation, still tend to give rather crucial shape to the patterns of hospital care.

My treatment of the themes, however, is obviously limited in quite another way (not intended in the dictionary definition). Most book introductions find the author acknowledging his or her limitations in insight, data, vision or whatever. Surely, all of that applies to me. However, in a sense my personal limitations are compounded by the fact that I am not continuously involved in medical care. As a seminary teacher and ethicist I do work closely with health care professionals in certain programs dealing with medicine and ethics. Nevertheless, the reader will recognize that the reflections in this volume are those of a concerned "allied professional" who does not, however, live daily within the hospital walls.

A second mark of the essay form is that it usually treats its subject from a personal point of view. In the following chapters I do not attempt to be neutral nor pretend to be unbiased. I have a viewpoint which I hope and believe is informed by the Christian faith. Readers who share that faith may find themselves at home with the theological language and imagery present in these pages. If, however, such religious language is unfamiliar and even appears to be out of place in the treatment of these issues, I urge you to consider several possibilities.

I urge you hold open the possibility that all of the topics addressed herein have very basic religious dimensions. I say this because I believe that people are essentially (and not accidentally) religious. Regardless of our formal church or synagogue affiliation, or lack thereof, our basic life attitudes and values are always based upon some sort of faith. That faith is the unprovable yet fundamental trust that certain things are real, worthwhile, important, worthy of our commitment, our energy, perhaps even our passion. And within that "faith stance" some center of value seems to be evident, some central reality, loyalty, or conviction around which other loyalties and values take their shape. In this broad yet basic way, life is inherently religious and, as part of life, medical care is, also. If you will grant this possibility, then it makes sense at least to inquire about the religious dimensions of the physician's identity or about the manner in which unprovable values give shape to our health care delivery.

I urge you, further, to be open to the religious dimension of these subjects, for medical care and the Christian religion have been inextricably intertwined in our social history. The late English physician-theologian Robert A. Lambourne frequently noted this in his writings. For example, in the primitive church the eucharist or sacramental meal was experienced principally as a communal sharing of new health and new life. Its focus was corporate, participatory, and positive. Only later did the eucharist become clericalized, individualized, and remedial. Then it was understood as an activity designed to eradicate specific defects (sins), and as an activity which the authorized clerical professional performed on behalf of the passive individual supplicant. The point is that in the "clinicalization" of modern medicine this pattern basically is reenacted. Medical care is seen primarily as the eradication of defects through technical processes defined and used by authorized professionals. A pattern of church practice contributed to the shaping of medical practice. Surely, the pattern of influence has gone in the other direction as well: religious professionals in recent decades have been strongly influenced in their own professional identities by a therapeutic medical model. Thus, the influence goes in both directions, and the histories are intertwined. Without raising some religious questions, we cannot understand modern medicine.

Finally and most importantly, I believe that a theologically informed approach to issues surrounding the person in medical care is warranted because, at their best, the aims of the church's ministry and the ministrations of medical science converge. Both endeavors are concerned about the wholeness of persons—or, at their *best* moments are thus concerned. Surely the hospital uses different means than does the church. There are also differences in the perceptions of ends to be sought. But, as those readers who are intimately involved in both church and hospital well know, the healing of the whole person is paramount to both groups and each needs the other. It is, after all, no historical accident that "health" and "salvation" come from the same linguistic root. For these several reasons, then, I believe it important to look at the person in medical care not only from humanistic perspectives but also from the theological.

There is a third reason for using the term. Essays are relatively short analytic or interpretive pieces, usually written to stand by themselves rather than as integral pieces of a larger composition. Such is true of the origin of five of the seven chapters of this book. The major themes of these five chapters took shape in addresses to different groups, even though a common thread binds them together. In revising them for this volume I have intentionally left some of the characteristics of oral address intact, so that a reasonably informal and conversational atmosphere might be present. It is my hope that these thoughts will contribute to the ongoing conversation about these matters.

The groups for whom portions of the following were written have my sincere thanks for their hospitality and their openness to dialog: The Manitoba Health Congress, Winnipeg; The National Association of Health and Welfare Ministries, New Orleans; The Synod of Lakes and Prairies, United Presbyterian Church, St. Paul; United Theological Seminary Convocation, New Brighton, Minnesota; Upper Midwest Hospital Conference, St. Paul; University of Minnesota Medical School Commencement, Minneapolis; University of Wisconsin Continuing Education Conference, Madison; and the West Virginia University School of Medicine Commencement, Morgantown. In addition, I am grateful to the editors of two publications in which earlier versions of Chapters II and V were subsequently printed: *Medical Bulletin,* University of Minnesota (Summer, 1974), and *Theological Markings,* United Theological Seminary of the Twin Cities, Vol. 44, No. 1 (Spring, 1974).

My seminary and family partners-in-concern receive my continuous gratitude and celebration for being part of them. I am grateful also to good friends and colleagues at the Program in Human Sexuality, University of Minnesota Medical School. And my thanks, once again, to Elsie Johnson for her skillful typing.

Finally, I want to record a special word to three staff members of Hennepin County Medical Center, Minneapolis: Ronald E. Cranford, M.D., Chaplain James A. Anderson, and Chaplain Lloyd E. Beebe. For stimulating collegiality in medical ethics classes, for manuscript suggestions, and especially for caring friendship, I thank you.

United Theological Seminary   J.B.N.
  of the Twin Cities

1

Underlying Issues
in the
Biomedical Debates

Regardless of whether one is a medical professional or a medical layperson, the complexity of current biomedical discussions makes it rather easy to succumb to the Charlie Brown syndrome. One of Schulz's classic "Peanuts" strips pictured the three children lying on their backs on a grassy slope, gazing at the clouds in the summer sky. Said Lucy, "If you use your imagination, you can see lots of things in the cloud formations . . . What do you think you see, Linus?" "Well," began Linus, "those clouds up there look to me like the map of the British Honduras on the Caribbean . . . That cloud up there looks a little like the profile of Thomas Eakins, the famous painter and sculptor . . . And that group of clouds over there gives me the impression of the stoning of Stephen . . . I can see the Apostle Paul standing there to one side . . ." Obviously approving this response, Lucy then turned to her now-wide-eyed second companion. "What do *you* see in the clouds, Charlie Brown?" Came the hapless reply, "Well, I was going to say I saw a ducky and a horsie, but I changed my mind." [1]

Faced with the technical and ethical entanglements of artificial inovulation and the artificial heart our first responses might indeed sound like "a ducky and a horsie," though hopefully a more careful examination of these and other problems would produce more Linus-like sophistication. But it is not the primary purpose of this book to examine such problems as these, important as they are. Other volumes usefully do that.[2] Rather, our primary focus is on the persons who are involved in making the day-to-day decisions about health care—patients and their families, physicians and nurses, hospital chaplains and parish ministers, citizens and special interest groups.

The problem areas themselves are of far-reaching importance, and perhaps it is understandable that thus far they have received the lion's share of attention in biomedical ethics. But it is also important that we understand more clearly the persons who are both the subjects and shapers of particular medical decisions. After all, what I intentionally do in a given situation is determined not only by my beliefs and values, the circumstances of the situation, and the available options. What I do is also molded by my own sense of identity in that situation and by my perception and understanding of other persons who are involved.[3]

Before we look more directly at the personhood of those (including ourselves) involved in medical decision-making, consider why the whole scope of "medical ethics" has changed dramatically. Only a generation ago, medical ethics was largely a concern of the physician alone. The subject dealt primarily with matters of etiquette—basic courtesies among doctors, the relationship of doctor and patient, and a few matters of medical jurisprudence. But three developments caused all this to change.

First there was the virtual explosion in sophisticated medical technology beginning in the 1950s and gaining momentum in the next two decades. Whether we are considering the moral issues surrounding death and dying or organ transplantation or abortion or the new genetics or the just distribution of health care, the rapid advances in medical technique are a vital part of the context. And through the mass media the public has become informed and has exhibited a lively interest in each new development.

These technological break-throughs came in the wake of another factor: the atrocities committed by Nazi physicians upon Jews and prisoners of war had raised to world consciousness the significant difference between basic moral issues and matters of mere etiquette.[4] The wide-spread revulsion against these acts led to the Nurenberg Code of Ethics for the health professions, later to the Helsinki Declaration, and then to the Geneva revision of the Hippocratic Oath subsequently adopted by the United Nations. It had become apparent that substantive moral issues increasingly faced modern medicine.

A third impetus to broadening the scope of medical ethics was a society increasingly concerned about the quality of life. Experiences of the past two decades convinced a great many Americans that preoccupation with quantity was simply not enough. There was a tragic war. There were shocking assassinations. Liberation movements arose. Minorities raised their claims for social justice with new power. A sense of urgency about world hunger and population began to develop. Awareness of ecological issues grew. A crisis of confidence in those who govern us occurred. In each of these experiences we were confronted by the quality questions: what quality of life do we now have? what do we want? what quality of life ought we rightfully have?

Hence, the whole scope of medical ethics changed. No longer a subject of concern to medical professionals alone, no longer a restricted matter of interpersonal etiquette and legal obligation, it became a subject for all of us, for none would be left untouched by its problems and its possibilities.

There are a number of underlying issues which weave their way in and out of each of the problem areas in medical ethics. These issues are both ethical and theological, and they seem to be present whether one is considering the discontinuance of medical supports for a terminally-ill patient, whether one is considering the use of artificial insemination, or whether one is reflecting on any of the host of other medical possibilities now before us. I believe that five such issues are of particular importance: (1) facts and values; (2) the "human" and the "personal"; (3) health and wholeness; (4) the individual and the society; and (5) the Creator and the creature.

Each of these issues is significant in the way that it makes connections between the medical problem and the persons in the midst of the decision. My treatment of them will reflect my own Christian orientation, which will be evident throughout this book. Hopefully, however, the reader who does not share this faith orientation will find numerous points of common ground with a writer convinced that it is God's purpose to nurture the fullest possible personal humanity of all people and that this process of humanization is effected through persons of widely differing faith persuasions as well as through those who claim none.

Facts and Values

First, there is a real difference between facts and values. The values of human life have not appeared more clearly just because we now have more accuracy about the facts of life. For example, simply because we have an enormously augmented understanding of the manner of the brain's functioning does not mean that we know any more about what is worthwhile in life. Knowledge of what *is* is important, indeed; but knowledge of what is will never tell us what *ought* to be.

The facts-values difference is nowhere more dramatically illustrated than in the debate over the definition of death. This debate has been occasioned, of course, by advances in medical technology. Not many years ago, all of us—physician and layperson alike—were sure we knew what death was: when spontaneous respiration and heartbeat ceased, the individual was dead. Nowadays, death as a *process* has become common medical currency. When respiration and heartbeat cease, there is clinical death; but sometimes resuscitation can reverse clinical death. When it is not reversed, brain death begins to occur. First the higher brain capacities controlling consciousness die, followed by the lower brain capacities governing primitive reflexes and vital functions, particularly respiration. Thereafter, biological death follows, the permanent extinction of bodily life, followed by the death of the body's cells in varying degrees.

About the *facts* of this process, there is agreement. But just when in the course of this process is the individual truly dead? The moral questions arise, of course, in regard to the use of heroic or extraordinary medical means to prolong life (or to prolong the dying process, as the case may be). But the advent of organ transplantation also pointedly raises the value questions. Scientifically we know that certain organs can be transplanted from a dead individual to a recipient. We also know that the cadaver donor must not be "so dead" that physical deterioration has made the kidney or heart useless for the transplant. We know *scientifically* when removal of the organs is still viable. But when is the removal *morally* viable? That is a different question.

A few years ago, a distinguished committee was assembled at Harvard under the leadership of Dr. Henry K. Beecher. It was called the Ad Hoc Committee of the Harvard Medical School to Examine the Definition of Brain Death. Their published report was entitled "A Definition of Irreversible Coma," and it began with this sentence: "Our primary purpose is to define irreversible coma as a new criterion for death."[5] Immediately the facts and values question is before us.[6] It is one thing to undertake the medical task of developing criteria for the prediction of irreversible coma or brain death. It is quite another thing to say that brain death equals human death. The former is an empirical task, a question of scientific fact. The latter is an ethical, philosophical, and theological task, a question of human value. In its original report the committee did not clearly distinguish the two questions. It was only in subsequent reflection that committee members acknowledged that their report was basically a scientific definition of irreversible coma, and that they would recommend that such coma be taken as a sign of death.

To say that irreversible coma *equals* death is to make a judgment based upon certain non-medical, non-scientific assumptions about what is essentially constitutive of human life. And what essentially constitutes human life is a philosophical and theological question about which medical professionals have every right and duty to voice their convictions but for which their medical training gives them no particular expertise. Thus, there is a "leap of faith" which divides fact questions from value questions. Given a certain definition of death, the establishment of criteria and the application of those criteria in *knowing when death has occurred* is a scientific and medical task. It is a fact question. But the *definition* of death is not a scientific question for the medical professionals; it is a human question for all of us.

Here is the victim of a tragic accident, lying in the intensive care unit of the hospital. Extensive brain damage has been sustained in the accident, and the electro-encephalogram (EEG) traces a flat line: no evidence of brain activity and no medical hope for recovery of such. Yet, the respirator with its regular wheeze continues to activate the lungs and circulate the blood. Are we dealing here with a living human being who still makes moral claims upon us to continue the best in care at whatever cost to family and society? Or are we dealing here with an unburied corpse, some of whose biological functions are being artificially maintained? The scientific facts will not answer that question. The question has become a matter of value, indeed of ultimate faith. What is the life which God the Creator has given us and calls us to guard, enhance, and care for? And what is the meaning of a resurrection faith in the Redeeming God, that faith which might save us from biological idolatries and from insisting upon the continuation of physical existence, regardless of its quality, at any price? The value questions are ultimately faith questions. They are never answered by medical facts alone, however sophisticated that medical knowledge and technique has become.

Human and Personal

Already we have begun to deal with the second question: the question of human and personal.[7] What does it mean to be "human"? We use the adjective in many different ways. We use it in a negative sense to point to our frailty, particularly moral frailty, our feet of clay. "After all, I'm only human—what did you expect, perfection?" Or, as a seasoned old Jesuit priest once wrote, "All things human, given enough time, go badly." But we also use the adjective "human" in a positive sense. We use it to describe that quality of existence which somehow ought to characterize our lives. "There," we say of an admired person, "goes an example of real humanity."

It is in this second and positive sense that the question—what does it mean to be human?—underlies the whole range of medical issues today. As we have already seen, the question hovers over the dying process: when are we prolonging human life, and when are we only prolonging a biological existence which has ceased to be meaningfully and recognizably human? The question is ever-present in the abortion issue: when are we dealing with a bit of tissue, and when are we dealing with a human being in the uterus? The question pervades the areas of genetic control, of transplant surgery, of sex-change operations, and a host of others: when are we promoting authentically human existence?

Again, it is a faith question, a theological one. The writer of the 8th Psalm addressed the issue (albeit in exclusively masculine language), asking: "What is man that thou art mindful of him, and the son of man that thou dost care for him?" The Psalmist answered his question with the affirmation that, paradoxically, human beings are similar to both God and the lower animal. Like God and unlike the animal, we are *free*. We have the capacity for self-transcendence; we are spirit; we are not limited to the animal's instinctual choices; we can remember our past, write our histories, contemplate our futures, project ourselves into the not-yet. Thus, if we are gifted with freedom, every medical procedure which violates our freedom, which simply treats us as objects of manipulation, which assumes that others must decide what quality of life is good for us, will dehumanize us.

Yet, unlike God and like the animal, reminds the Psalmist, we are also *finite*. Our Creator has given boundaries to our lives; we have been given death as well as birth. Hence, every medical procedure which violates our finitude (assuming, for example, that continued bodily existence, regardless of the quality of life, is to be sought at all costs) is also dehumanizing.

And, as Reinhold Niebuhr so often reminded us, because we human beings live on that dizzy pinnacle between freedom and finitude, participating in both but fearing to embrace both dimensions of our lives fully, we are anxious and our lives are filled with ambiguity. Hence, we do well to remember that all of our significant medical decisions are ambiguous. They are never simply black or white, never as clear-cut as we would like to think or hope. But those decisions are also potentially meaning-filled.

Another way of pointing to our essential humanity is to say that we are religious beings. We are fated with being inherently religious—everyone is, whether he or she consciously professes a religious faith or not. That is, we are so made that we must seek meaning, ultimate meaning, for our personal and social existence. And we find that meaning in relatedness—in the capacity to respond to other persons and to God.

Our relatedness as social beings is not only with others, but within ourselves as well, for we are multi-dimensional in our humanness. We are not merely body, nor merely soul. We are not merely mechanisms, nor compounds of chemicals, nor psychological existences. We are all of these systems and processes, seeking integration and creative unity. And if so, genuinely humanizing medicine must treat more than one part of the individual; it must care for the whole self.

All of these comments about what constitutes the "human" quality of our lives strongly suggest a companion term: the *personal* quality. That which concerns us is not simply biologically human life, but even more the capacity for personal human life: the lives of beings who are both finite and free, who are relational and social in their existence, who are seeking for meaning, who can commit themselves to causes. Our mandate is to preserve and enhance not only genetically human life as such, but also and even more importantly we are to enhance personal human life. It is a relative, risky, ambiguous distinction, to be sure. It is also one which is terribly necessary.

If you are willing to make that distinction, the abortion question is never automatically answered by asserting that we are dealing with human life *in utero*. Of course we are, and that human life is precious. And during pregnancy as that pre-personal human life gradually acquires increased personal potentiality, its claims upon us become ever more weighty. If in fetal life we encounter pre-personal humanity, in the irreversibly comatose patient we encounter post-personal human life. It is still a valued human life, but the moral claims upon us are different when personhood has been permanently extinguished. All created life is precious in God's sight and is to be valued by us, but personhood lays upon us its particular moral claims.

Health and Wholeness

The third pervasive issue in medical ethics today is the meaning of health and wholeness. What is health? Interestingly and significantly, our dictionaries tend to define health in negative, individualistic, and partial ways—ways which reflect our common cultural understandings. We think of health negatively, as freedom from disease or defect. We think of health individualistically, as a condition of the individual person. We think of health partially and functionally, as dealing with isolated parts and functions of our bodies.[8]

But notice how these accents in our definition of health both fail to do justice to more biblical notions and also lead to certain practical results. When our understandings are more negative than positive, we emphasize curing diseases much more than we emphasize maintaining health. This is reflected in our allocation of financial and social acclaim: in the medical profession it is the surgeon who commands the highest income and prestige, while the physician in public health and preventive medicine receives lesser rewards. But a more biblical view would have us see health positively—as caring for human wholeness.

We think of health individualistically. Of course it is true that health has to do with the individual. The biblical perspective, however, reminds us that we are social and relational beings. What individual can be healthy when that person's social or natural environment is polluted?

We tend to think of health partially and functionally. But health involves wholeness, and that which treats only part of me may still leave me unhealed. The growth of a cancer may require surgery, the mechanical removal of a diseased part of my body. But healing in one dimension does not necessarily bring healing in other dimensions of my personhood. I am more than a biological machine, and repair of one of my parts will not necessarily overcome my fragmentation.

Thus, a richer view of health invites us to cure human diseases, yes, but even more fundamentally to care for human health in the positive sense of human well-being. The World Health Organization (WHO) some years ago articulated this in its now well-known definition: "Health is a state of complete physical, mental, and social well-being and not merely the absence of disease or infirmity." Later in this book we shall examine some of the problems implicit in the WHO definition. At this point, however, I wish to emphasize its positive contributions to our re-thinking of the meaning of health.

The first virtue of the WHO definition is its recognition that any definition of health is value-laden. Health is not a neutral, scientific concept, pure and simple. It reflects the values of those who shape it. In this instance it reflects the conviction of WHO that health is a positive state of human well-being and fulfillment.

Second, "it is a definition which implies that there is some intrinsic relationship between the good of the body and the good of the self." [9] There is no dualism of the self and the body here. The person is recognized as a whole being. If one drops a brick on the toe, this is not simply an experience of the body; it also concentrates the mind and emotions wonderfully.

A further virtue is that this positive definition of health is an ideal. It points to how things ought to be. The norm is an ideal of complete wholeness. Any definition of health describes the state of persons in relation to some concept of normality. If the definition is one of pathology (a negative definition), then health is the absence of diseases or impairments which are defined as pathological. If the norm of health is a statistical one, normality takes its form from the modal distribution of qualities in a population. Thus, if the majority of people are of a certain shape and weight, of a certain physio-emotional balance, and of a certain range of intellectual ability, then obesity, hypertension, and mental deficiency find their definitions as illnesses by deviating too markedly from that norm. While there are values bound up with each of these ways of describing normality, the WHO definition is distinguished by positing an ideal. True, that ideal is unattainable and imprecise. But, as physician Mervyn Susser wisely states, "there is more danger in encouraging the fallacy that what can only be narrowly measured must also be narrowly conceived, than in aspiring to measure or attain an ideal. . . . To accept less is to support the status quo, a not uncommon position for the health professions despite their avowed altruism and implicit reformism." [10]

Finally, the WHO definition of health solidly links the individual with his or her community. It embraces a notion of *social* well-being. And that leads to the next of the pervasive, underlying issues in medical ethics.

Individual and Society

The fourth theme which threads its way through virtually all medical ethics problems today is the ancient issue of the individual and the society. One way in which this issue can be seen is in the style of decision-making itself. It is the old question of "ethics of right" in contrast with "ethics of good." What is the appropriate emphasis in making our decisions? Shall we decide basically in terms of the rights of the individual and of our duties toward that person? Or rather shall we pay more attention to the consequences of the various medical options before us, calculating the morality of the act according to the greatest good or widest social benefits which might be achieved by the decision?

Individual rights or the good of society? For example, are the rights of a married couple sacrosanct in their choices about having children? Should others never interfere with those rights? But what if the couple are carriers of a genetic disease? Should that couple be allowed to procreate even if society must bear the main burden of caring for a grossly-deformed child?

Individual rights or social benefits? The issue is pointedly present in the ethics of experimenting with human subjects. A few years ago, Dr. Saul Krugman of Willowbrook Hospital in New York experimented with a group of institutionalized, mentally-retarded children. With the knowledge and consent of their parents, he deliberately infected each child in the control group with a mild case of hepatitis, a serious liver disease. Commenting on this case, a nationally-known physician noted that while there was a tremendous uproar over the ethics of this experiment, the end results were fantastic, and they couldn't have been obtained without using human subjects.

What do we say to this? The sturdy defender of an ethics of the right and of protection of the individual person will say that this type of experimentation is simply wrong. Regardless of how much good might come to future generations, no parents have the right to give consent for a medical experiment which has no possible therapeutic benefit for their child. No parent ought to consent and no parent ought even be asked. And no doctor has the right deliberately to induce disease into children like this. It is intrinsically and fundamentally wrong.[11]

There are others, also thoughtful and sensitive persons, who think differently. In ethics generally and in biomedical research especially it is much more appropriate to reason inductively from the specific data of the particular situation than to conclude a priori that whole classes of actions are inherently right or wrong. What really counts is good results, and results are good when they add up to a net gain for human well-being. In any human experimentation there will be some risk to those involved, but if those risks are carefully controlled they should be taken for the future benefit of countless people yet unborn.[12]

We need both of these emphases. If our only focus is upon the wider social benefit of medical experimentation, then we open the doors once again to the brutalities of Nazi experimental medicine in Germany of the 1930s and 1940s. We open the doors once again to the brutalities of our own American publicly-funded 30-year experiment on 400 black men who were deceived by government doctors so that the experimenters could observe the effects of untreated syphilis.

But we also need concern about the wider society and about future generations. There is moral harm in not doing research as well as risk in doing it. We need concern about both ends and means, both present and future, both individual and society. Our overarching responsibility is to God. God is the One who values each individual person beyond all human valuing, and also the One who calls us into the risks of moral ambiguity to increase the good of wider society and of generations yet unborn.

If the individual-society issue is always present in the style of our decision-making, it is also present in the closely-related matter of our basic stance toward medical care. Our Western society is heir to a strong philosophic and cultural tradition of individualism, and that tradition remains particularly potent in the United States. Individualism as a basic orientation wears many faces, but several underlying ideas are common to its different expressions: the supreme value and dignity of the individual human being; the right of each person to autonomy in making his or her own significant decisions; the right to privacy and freedom from interference by the wider community in one's most significant activities; the high emphasis upon self-development for each individual; and the notion that the individual is the central reality while community, society, and the state are of secondary importance and reality.[13]

In biomedical ethics we frequently find apparently contradictory attitudes about such individualism. On the one hand, it seems to be the source of many of our difficulties in current medical care. We are unclear about what it means. (The person defending, on grounds of the right to "privacy," the right of any pregnant woman desiring an abortion to have one, is often the same person who resists the use of the individual privacy argument by those who would exclude minority groups from their neighborhoods.) Furthermore, while the rhetoric of individualism is all around us, we seem tongue-tied in terms of language of the public good. The language of medical individualism results in a one-to-one contract model for dispensing medical care, creating problems of finding appropriate therapy for those who can afford it and excluding those who cannot. As such, it is insufficient.

However, there is much in individualism that we want to protect. We rightly fear the possibilities for social control which inhere in some of the new biotechnologies. We seek to preserve and augment individual freedoms and the personal therapeutic relationships in our search for better ways of distributing medical care. Thus, the individual-society issue pervades every nook and cranny of biomedical ethics today.

Creator and Creature

All of this leads to the fifth basic issue underlying these medical areas: Creator and creature. Shall we "play God"? Surely it is basic to the Judeo-Christian faith that creatures should not confuse themselves with the Creator. Idolatry results and human suffering ensues when people play God. In medical matters, simply because we have the technological capacity to do certain things does not mean that we are morally justified in doing them. We may or may not be.

But the notion of playing God becomes very confusing—and I believe that it is confused by essentially unbiblical notions about both God and human nature. Think, for example, of typical responses we often hear in discussions about death and dying: if we intervene in the dying process, we have wrongly allowed human decisions to affect the time and manner of the individual's

death, but if we allow the disease to take its course then we have
not usurped God's place and power. But that is a strange argument. If pushed to its logical conclusion it would prevent us from
using any kind of medical intervention at any stage in any disease. It would prevent any alteration of any natural process. Yet,
its advocates are usually more selective than that. They are like
the 85-year-old midwestern grandmother whose birthday gift
from her children was a ticket for her first plane ride—to visit
relatives in California. After refusing the ticket with the familiar
words, "If God had wanted us to fly, God would have given us
wings," she added, "No, sir, I'll just sit here and watch my nice
color TV like the good Lord intended!"

There is a long theological history behind our confusions about
Creator and creature.[14] In addition to the essentially Christian
insight about God's nature—a personal, loving God—we also
inherit ways of seeing God as an impersonal, coercive force or
power. But we can't have it both ways. If God's central nature
is personal love, then God is not a puppet-master pulling the
strings. God is not the naked power of a machine, but rather the
persuasiveness of personality. Not force, but lure and attraction.
Not coercion but intentionality. God rules not through the impo-
sition of arbitrary and static laws, but rather through an intimate
relationship to and participation in the events of the world.
Luther saw it rightly: "God rules, yes, but God rules from
a cross."

There is also a long theological history to our views about the
human creature. We are influenced not only by the biblical notions of humanity, but also by the Greco-Roman vision of natural
law. When Christians in the early centuries of the church tried
to combine these two visions of humanness, they were living and
thinking in a pre-scientific, non-technological, agrarian society.
There they were developing a rather detailed notion of what was
proper to human nature (in other words, what was in accord
with natural law) and what was not. For example, to the Christian of centuries ago, the cutting out of a healthy organ from a
healthy person's body was a grave sin against natural law and

against nature's God. To the Christian living in the era of organ transplants, this might be a high act of self-giving love.

Thus, our notions about what it means to play God have changed, or at least they should change. If we believe in a static, unchanging deity who is removed from involvement in our world and who has pre-ordained certain strict limits to what human nature is and how it should express itself, that is one thing. But if we believe in the God whose name is Cosmic Love, who is involved, rejoicing, and suffering in the midst of the created world, who is luring persons toward greater fulfillment of their intended humanity, who is allowing them freedom to grow and create—then that is another vision of Creator and creature. We are, indeed, called to "play God" if that means responsible participation as co-creators in what humankind is yet to be.

Thus, it is extremely difficult to draw hard and fast lines in many of these issues. We need to weigh carefully the whole range of new biomedical procedures in all of their promise and all of their ambiguity. For example, are sperm banks for artificial human insemination a violation of God's natural order? Is artificial insemination all right for cattle, but have we crossed the fateful line when we use that technique for human procreation? Neither a simple yes or no answer is adequate. For a stable, child-desiring couple rendered infertile by the husband's sterility, artificial insemination might be a gracious and humanizing possibility. But used on a massive scale (as some have proposed) as an attempt to improve the genetic quality of the human race, it would appear far more threatening than promising for human personhood.

To open ourselves to co-creativity with God—to "play God" in the positive sense of the word—ought not to blind us to our human finitude and sin. We need to remember that there is both a grandeur and a misery about human nature. We are capable of noble acts and selfless moral wisdom. We are also prone to our ego-trips, our selfish and distorted judgments. There is room, at one and the same time, for both optimism and pessimism about ourselves, and that is a hopeful Christian realism.

A hopeful realism can go far in counteracting the extreme scenarios of technological utopias, on the one hand, and nightmarish doomsdays, on the other. We are neither at the mercy of mad scientists of comic-book variety, nor are we in the hands of the utterly wise and benevolent scientists who hold out the path of salvation for the race. Without any ingratitude for the brilliance of biomedical achievements, some of us still believe that ultimately our salvation lies beyond any human revolution, even the scientific one. So we are left with a more modest posture: rejoicing in the biomedical developments which contribute so much to the relief of human suffering and the enhancement of human fulfillment; weighing each new development carefully in all of its ambiguity; and putting it all in the focus of the eyes of faith—a faith which sees Creator and creature participating together in the task of humanizing life.

I suspect that Thornton Wilder captured something of this perspective in *Our Town,* a play from the thirties which still wears surprisingly well. He senses the uniqueness of each person while recognizing that each is part of a much wider society, and all of it in ultimate dimensions. The scene is that in which the children are talking about a letter:

REBECCA: I never told you about that letter Jane Crofut got from her minister when she was sick. . . . He wrote Jane a letter and on the envelope the address was like this: It said:

Jane Crofut — the Crofut Farm — Grover's Corners — Sutton County—New Hampshire—United States of America.

GEORGE *(interrupting):* What's so funny about that?

REBECCA: But listen, it's not finished: the United States of America—Continent of North America—Western Hemisphere —the Earth—the Solar System—the Universe—the Mind of God—that's what it said on the envelope.

GEORGE: What do you know!

REBECCA: And the postman brought it just the same.

GEORGE: What do you know! [15]

The Personhood
of the
Physician

The Changing Medical Scene

At least some things in medicine have not changed very much. By the second half of the 1970s physicians' insurance rates had soared out of sight. Doctors' strikes had occurred. "Defensive medicine" was common, leaving no stone unturned even at the risk of overtesting and overtreating. The threat of punitive malpractice suits lay behind it all, and it all seemed very new. But those familiar with the history of medicine might recall these lines from the Code of Hammurabi, dating some 3600 years ago: "If a surgeon operates on a man . . . and the man gets well from a tumor or disease of the eye, the surgeon will receive ten silver shekels. . . . If the man dies because the tumor is cut or the destruction of his eye, then the surgeon's hands shall be cut off." Unfortunately, there are precedents to some of our painful contemporary problems.

But other things about medicine have obviously changed. Less than a hundred years ago, the physician carried in his head and his hands (it was almost always a "him") virtually everything he needed to treat his patients according to the knowledge and standards of the day. He charged about twenty-five cents for an office call (usually including medicine), and fifty to seventy-five cents for a house call. An obstetrics case brought the princely sum of five dollars. Hospital admissions were uncomplicated, and hospital treatment typically was handled by a single doctor.[1]

The changes today clearly are far greater than the changes in costs, dramatic as those may be. Already we have noted the astounding biomedical developments which have occurred. And the *New England Journal of Medicine* has no corner on the market in the discussion of these issues, for this month's *Reader's Digest* and this week's Sunday supplement most likely will carry articles on extraordinary life supports or transplants or the new genetics.

Future predictions are always risky. Will Rogers once said, with characteristic elegance, that those who insist upon gazing into the crystal ball should have that ball stuck into their mouths. Nevertheless, it takes little foresight to realize that the technological developments in medicine realized in the century's third quarter will undoubtedly continue and intensify. In addition, it now seems clear that new dimensions in medical change are upon us. During the fourth quarter these changes will come not only from the research laboratories, but also from the inner laboratories of experience wherein professional and personal identities are shaped.

Artists and Artisans

The physician's professional identity is intimately linked with his or her understanding of "the art of medicine." But, what is an art? The word in its basic meaning and linguistic ancestry signifies a skill or an ability. Yet skills and abilities can be directed to different types of ends. The dictionaries suggest that one may be designated either an artisan or an artist, depending upon whether one's skills are directed principally toward a utilitarian purpose or an aesthetic purpose. Thus, the artisan is the skilled craftsperson whose abilities are aimed at some tangible goal, some useful end. The artist, on the other hand, is primarily concerned with the imaginative communication of a perception of life's quality—its beauty, its reality, its intended form.

Ideally, the physician ought to be neither one nor the other but clearly both at once—consciously and conscientiously both artisan and artist. As artisan, the doctor is a skilled craftsperson exercising competence in the science of medicine: caution, exactitude, and careful clinical judgments. As artist, the doctor is forever conscious that quality-of-life issues are at stake and that cases are always persons with hopes and fears.

Priests and Prophets

The important internal professional tension between artisan and artist can be expanded and enriched by the use of two other polar terms from the imagery of religion: priest and prophet. In every major religion of the world we see these two types of religious leaders, and occasionally we see individuals in whom these two roles are combined in a remarkably creative way. The priestly orientation has (1) a strong ritual emphasis, (2) a strong focus on the individual, and (3) a tendency to affirm the institution within which the priestly activity goes on. In contrast, the prophetic orientation (1) focuses more on the ethical than on the ritualistic, (2) has a more social than individual focus, and (3) tends to engage in constructive institutional criticism.

Consider first the priest. Here is the one who is obviously the religious person in the society. Often identified by a special garb, the priest is the keeper of the temple. Here is the one who leads and understands the religious ritual in some depth. Here is the one whose ministry is oriented to the care of each individual in the congregation, the one whom parishioners trust and come to in times of need. Here is the professional caretaker of the religious institution. This is the priest.

Perhaps this religious imagery is not so far-fetched when applied to the doctor. In fact, throughout most of the history of the West, the medical person was regarded as a priest and religious functionary.[2] Indeed, until the age of the Renaissance it was commonly assumed that diseases were either divinely or demonically caused. True, during the next three hundred years the religiosity of medicine declined, for by then it was too late in the development of human thought to blame God for diseases but still too early for medical science to work its own wonders. However, by the second quarter of this century, our high faith in science coupled with medicine's remarkable new abilities to cure disease combined to assure doctors of religious status once again, whether they wanted it or not.

Though the high priestly image of the physician is beginning to change, there is still considerable public sympathy for it. Occupational prestige? While the Harris Poll indicates that in the last ten years doctors have dropped more percentage points in prestige than any other profession, nevertheless the physician is still at the top as the most trusted of all professionals. Rewards? The average salary of the doctor still leads the list. The "generalization of expertise"? It is still there. Even though his or her professional training and schedule may permit little time for study of public issues, many people will still cast the doctor in the role of expert on every non-medical matter from school bond issues to foreign policy, simply because a doctor's opinions somehow ought to carry more weight than those of "the ordinary person."

Further, many a patient still finds the visit to the doctor something of a religious experience. The physician still usually wears a garment of white, which is not only a sign of clinical cleanliness but also seems to be a symbol of purity dividing the holy from the diseased. The doctor uses a technical language, and secret language always seems to possess cultic power. And consider the ritual which usually marks the clinic visit. When I am a patient, I confess my sin, I am assured of absolution, and I receive the prescription of penitential acts—a ritual whose ancient religiosity surely makes some imprint upon my subconscious mind. If all of this seems to be stretching things a bit, just pause and reflect: most people perceive the words of the clergy as "counsel," the words of their lawyer as "advice," but they perceive the words of their doctor as "orders" to be "religiously followed."

If the physician-priest image still dominates in our society, it is also changing. The voice of the prophet is heard in the land. The prophet is also religious, but in a rather unconventional way. Instead of emphasizing ritual, the prophet emphasizes the ethical. Instead of focusing simply on the individual, the prophet always sees the individual as part of a larger society, a society which stands in need of change. Not so much the keeper and the defender of the religious establishment, the prophet is engaged in a lover's quarrel with these institutions. Throughout our religious history, the prophet has appeared in many forms and guises. Some have been the ancient predecessors of the counter culture, appearing in hair shirts and eating locusts and wild honey. But others have worn their Brooks Brothers suits, or the equivalent thereof.

Look more closely at the prophet in the physician. A prophet is always religious but often appears to be secular. And we are beginning to see the secularization of the medical profession in our society. Whenever secularization occurs in any institution, it involves the voice and power of the laity challenging ultimate control by the professionals. The physician-prophet welcomes this challenge to medicine.

Remember that secularization began earlier in most other western institutions. The Reformations of the 16th century brought the process to the church (even though some clergy still forget that). Secularization came to the political state in the 18th and 19th centuries (though occasionally we still get political leaders who seem to believe in the divine right of kings). And in our own time, secularization has begun to affect medicine.

This process is never easy or comfortable for those who are most intimately affected. It calls for a rethinking of the inherited self-image. But it can also be very liberating, for an unqualified high priestly role belongs to no one—whether clergy or politician or corporation executive or physician. For the priestly role unchecked by the prophetic will diminish the humanity of those who assume it and endanger the humanity of those whom they try to serve.

The prophet does not resist the participation of the laity but rather welcomes it, knowing that while specialized knowledge is indeed the responsibility of the professional, the basic value decisions must be made in community. And the value choices are still very much with us in this last quarter century:

• the abortion controversy shows few signs of abating as yet, and it clearly is an ethical as well as a medical matter;

• what should or should not be done in prolonged terminal illness, and who should decide—these are questions which are still the daily agony of countless families as well as physicians;

• the awesome possibilities of genetic medicine are just now surfacing in the public forum, and they will affect our common future;

• the mounting costs of kidney dialysis will trigger new public debates about the allocation of scarce resources;

• the arguments over a national health care system will intensify;

• the coming of the totally-implantable artificial heart will open another chapter in the definition of death.

These issues and more like them in the coming years will continue to occupy the best in hard thinking and warm human compassion that physicians and public alike can muster. The physician-prophet welcomes the partnership, because these are matters of value choice for us all, and everyone has a stake in their outcome.

The Doctor's Inner Dialectic

The artisan-artist and the priest-prophet dimensions of the physician's identity can interweave and exist in a creative inner dialectic. As artist the physician always reaches beyond utilitarian competencies toward an imaginative communication of life's quality, its beauty, its human reality. If the artisan deals in analysis, objective facts, and general laws, the one who is also artist deals with feelings, with the drive toward wholeness, and with the uniqueness and particularity of subjects. The physician as artisan sees carcinoma and statistical prognosis. The physician as artist sees just as clearly the person with hopes and fears. Indeed, the commitment to care about persons with a moral artistry undergirds and often goes beyond the mandate to cure disease. As a wise physician has said, sometimes the doctor can cure, often the doctor can relieve pain, but always the doctor can care. Surely, when I am ill my need is for technically sophisticated therapy, but it goes beyond that. My human hunger is for one who gives personally to me—in terms of myself—not just technologically to me in terms of my defects. Genuine compassion (literally co-suffering, the ability of another to understand what my illness means to me) is neither pity nor paternalism, and it cannot be feigned. But when present it is unmistakably sensed by the patient.[3]

The physician's artistry thus is part of both the priestly and the prophetic dimensions of professional identity. There is an unmistakable artistry in caring for individual persons, a priestly task. There is also a prophetic moral artistry in dealing with decisional issues which go beyond the traditional codes. As noble and important as the Hippocratic Oath and its updated versions are, they are ethical starting points and not final answer books. There is no specific guidance therein for any of the new medical technologies, and no specific guidance for those situations in which basic principles come into conflict with each other (e.g. relieving suffering and prolonging life). But in practice the physician, even in the face of uncertainty, must act. Then moral artistry is called for. Good ethics, after all, is like good art. It is knowing where to draw the lines. And there is no canvas with lines already drawn and numbers inserted, for art is not painting by numbers nor is ethics prefabricated morality. Moral artistry is imaginative work on the canvas of human possibilities. Compassion is essential, but so also is disciplined and tough-minded grappling with fundamental human issues, a grappling which should take place in company with patient, family, and other members of the health care team.

In addition, the prophet sees not only the individual as focus for concern but knows that persons are inextricably bound up in the wider society. That the great ethical traditions of medicine have focused much more strongly upon the clinical relationship of the physician with the individual patient, there can be little doubt. The Hippocratic tradition is a noble base, but in this fourth quarter century, many physician-prophets see the need for creatively enlarging that base. Dr. Edmund Pellegrino, a noted medical educator, is one. He reminds us that the Hippocratic Oath enjoins the physician to work for patient benefit and to do no harm. Hippocrates' law sets out the requirements for competent medicine. His precepts deal with the need for consultations. And, says Dr. Pellegrino, what emerges is the picture of the doctor who is oriented primarily to the individual patient, a benign but authoritarian professional who is part of a secret brotherhood, who makes decisions in the best interest of the patient but who does not have a solid base for participatory medicine.[4] Another physician, Ivan Bennett, observed that "the inclination of many doctors to obstruct social change tends to make them strangers to the public and to colleagues with a greater social conscience."[5]

Indeed, the prophet-physicians are among us. It is indisputable, they tell us, that the United States has produced the best clinical and laboratory medicine in the world, and our quality of crisis care is second to none. It is also beyond reasonable doubt, they remind us, that in preventive medicine and in the maintenance of health, in longevity statistics and infant mortality, we suffer by comparison to many other industrialized nations. Prophets always remind us of the dispossessed. They remind us that lest compassion lose its wider vision and erode into sentimentality, compassion must mate with justice for the powerless inhabitants of the world. The physician-prophets among us are reminding us that serious questions about our health care system must be raised if the victims of racism or geography, age or income, educational deficit or social stigma are going to hope for a healthier day. They remind us of the interdependence of poverty and illness—the poor are much more likely to be chronically ill and the chronically ill are much more likely to be poor. They remind us that among the middle class, catastrophic and terminal illness care continues to destroy financially too many families. They remind us that rat bites, lead poisoning, napalm burns, Tay-Sachs disease, lung cancer, and starvation are not resolved simply by attending to the individual patient. Of all these things the prophet-physicians are painfully aware and will not let us forget.

We are reaching for an understanding of how the priestly and the prophetic can be combined in the individual physician. What might the model be? Surely the doctor's alternative is not simply the role of an applied scientist, an engineering model which makes the patient into a case and the doctor into a plumber. Nor is the alternative a simplistic affirmation of radical equality between physician and patient, which denies the very real and important functional differences between them. Nor is it simply the role of social reformer in which the professional can lose the zeal for high standards of clinical competence and integrity. Yet there is an alternative which, thankfully, many physicians are now embracing: that image of the colleague who possesses special competence.[6] This professional self-image invites new possibilities of trust and confidence with patients, for patients know that they are neither forced to nor will they be allowed to abdicate their own freedom in significant choices about their own futures. It is a self-image through which physicians increasingly welcome the public into partnership in setting medical priorities and resource allocation. It is a self-understanding through which physicians find criticism of the medical profession by others less personally threatening and less of an affront to their status.

A Different Medical Student?

The changes now occurring in physician identity can be understood further through a look at what is happening in the medical school's socialization process. One of the leading sociologists of medicine, Dr. Renee Fox, has studied the contrasts between

medical education in the 1950s and that of the 1970s. "Medical
education in the 1950s," she observes, "was more tightly and uni-
formly organized than it is now. Looking at it from the perspective of the 1970s, the medical school curriculum was arranged in
a 'lock-step' way, with little room for individual variation or
choice." [7] The first two years were dominated by lecture hall
presentations and laboratory work in pre-clinical and basic sciences, with minimal patient contact. As third and fourth year
students crossed over the great divide into clinical work, their
characteristic styles of dress symbolized the change. Long white
laboratory coats worn over khaki pants and sports shirts gave
way to short white coats, neckties, pressed trousers, new little
black bags, and stethoscopes hanging conspicuously out of the
white coat pockets. The 1950s' typical medical school curriculum
was a carefully-planned sequence, not only of content learning
but also of attitude socialization tasks. The student was to be
shaped with the proper balance of uncertainty and certainty, of
concern and detachment, of teamwork and individual initiative.
The medical school and hospital community of students and
teachers was assumed to be the appropriate and self-enclosed
world in which proper attitudes and self-images were to be
developed.

Medical education in the 1970s has been characterized by some
markedly different qualities. There is some evidence that a new
type of medical student is present. The percentage of women in
student bodies has increased, as has the percentage of racial and
ethnic minorities. There is some evidence that the typical student
is more "socially concerned, critical of the way that health care
is organized and delivered in American society (particularly to
the disadvantaged), determined to practice a more equitable,
feeling, and less driven medicine than his (or her) elders, and
committed to actively reforming medicine in ways that he (or
she) hopes will be ramified in nonmedical sectors of the society." [8]

Curricular organization and emphases have changed. Elective
and free time have been expanded. There is a new accent on programs in community medicine, social medicine, preventive medi-

cine, and family medicine. Fieldwork and practicum experience outside the walls of academic medical centers have increased considerably. Greater emphasis upon the relevance of the behavioral sciences and medical ethics is being felt.

Beyond these more observable changes in curricular structures, there are some interesting changes in the professional formation or attitude socialization process in the contemporary medical school. Faculty members seem more reluctant to be held accountable for the shaping of beliefs, attitudes, and conduct of the new generation of physicians. And students themselves seem more ambivalent in their attitudes toward their instructors. "As compared with their counterparts in the 1950s, students now tend to view their teachers as negative role models, not necessarily with rancor or disesteem but more as a symbolic expression of their resolve to be 'different,' 'better,' more socially responsible physicians than the medical 'establishment' with which they identify their instructors." [9]

It would be easy to overdraw this portrait of change in the medical student. In spite of recruiting efforts aimed at democratizing the constitution of the student body, the current medical student is still likely to be white, middle class, and male. He is still likely to trim his hair and his beard and to put on a tie when he begins to see patients. But it is safe to say that the new medical student is more likely than the student of twenty years ago to be staunchly egalitarian in his or her understanding of the doctor and the doctor's relationship to patients and non-physician members of the health care team. The new student is more likely to disapprove of all-knowing or omnipotent attitudes on the part of the doctor. The new student recognizes that some degree of objectivity toward the patient is necessary, but the "detached concern" model of some years ago is looked on with considerable suspicion by a new breed who place much higher value on feeling with the patient. It is also safe to say that there is considerably more emphasis on the physician's mandate to be more than just "a good human being," for the new medical student is more inclined toward concern with the meaning of life and death, suffering and corporate justice, issues basic both to the medical profession and to the human condition. If the 1950s seemed to many of us to be a remarkably clean-cut and wholesome period—filled with those of us reared on Walt Disney, Shirley Temple, the Scouts, and Juicy Fruit gum—perhaps the late 1970s, for all their ambiguity, pain, and moral untidiness, show some distinct signs of hope.

The hope is that the more prophetic dimensions of professional identity are being captured, to be held in creative tension with the priestly. Along with the ritual focus there is a new growth of the ethical. Along with the individual, the social. Along with institutional affirmation, the willingness to engage in institutional critique. It is a very uneven process, to be sure. Perhaps the majority of middle-aged and older practitioners will continue to see themselves more heavily in the priestly mold, and many will resent the changing expectations of their younger colleagues and of the patients and public. So, the professional identity perplexities are numerous. But the tensions of change are creative and hopeful.

The priestly and the prophetic dimensions of identity need each other. The priest who is not also prophet will find that priesthood increasingly barren in its ritual, individualistic rather than personal in its focus, and defensive about present institutions in a way that finally subverts the institutions themselves. It is true in organized religion and true in medicine as well.

Two Dimensions of "Graceful Identity"

Theologically speaking, both the priestly and the prophetic exist by the grace of God. In the Christian tradition there are two major motifs for expressing that grace: justification and sanctification. The symbol of justification by grace points to the faith that God's powerful love is infinitely greater than we can understand or deserve, and yet that undeserved acceptance is freely given. The symbol of sanctification points to the conviction that God's loving power can also be experienced by and expressed through human lives. Like the prophetic and the priestly, both justification and sanctification need each other in creative tension if we are to symbolize most adequately the meaning of God's love.

To this point in history, the tradition of medicine has clearly emphasized (albeit in largely secular terms) sanctification, the "holiness" of the practitioner. Early Hindu medical writings focused on the personal character, demeanor, and appearance of the physician—with emphasis on cleanliness, trimmed hair, neat clothes, and clean fingernails. Early Moslem medical treatises had similar emphases: the physician should not drink in public, should chew well while eating, should wear well-tailored clothes, and should remove excess hair from the face and head.[10] Percival's *Medical Ethics,* which is the immediate progenitor of American medical codes, is a treatise on "the Gentleman Physician." This, to be sure, is not simply an exhortation to be a polite and considerate doctor with *savoir faire,* but, in the 18th century meaning of "gentleman," to be a *virtuous* individual.[11]

Such sanctificationist concerns for both the decorum and personal virtue of the physician were not out of place in the ancient world or in the 18th century. Nor are they today. But when emphasis on sanctification is not balanced by justification, there result not only theological problems but also human distortions. Justification by grace has always reminded Christians that people can never be perfect, strive as they might; that we live creatively by acknowledging our limitations and failures as well as by trying to overcome them; that we are accepted because of God's infinite love and not because of our achievements.

There is a rough but meaningful correlation between a recovery of the reality of justification (whether expressed in traditional, modern, or even secular terms) and the growth of more prophetic medical professionals. The sanctificationist experience, important and necessary though it be, without its justificationist counterpart will always nurture high priests convinced of their own virtue and authority. With the reality Christianly symbolized as justification, however, comes also a healthy humility and the security necessary for professional and institutional critical self-examination. With it comes likewise the freedom to risk expressing the prophetic side of one's professional identity. It is as true for the medic as for the cleric. And the realities of "graceful identity" are not confined only to those physicians who perceive themselves through the language of the Christian tradition. Those who speak of these things in secular terms may well know their meaning.

3

The Personhood of the Chaplain

The favorite story of a Catholic friend of mine concerns the mother of a large family who was speaking to her priest one Sunday following mass. "That was a beautiful sermon you preached today on the joys of holy matrimony, Father," she said. Then the woman added, as if on second thought, "If I knew as little about it as you do, I think I could be as eloquent myself!" In addressing the personhood of the hospital chaplain I run a risk similar to that involved in speaking about the physician. It may seem presumptuous for one who is neither physician nor chaplain to write about these identity issues. Yet, these reflections come from an empathetic outsider who has benefitted immensely from close working relationships and friendships in these two professional groups.

Priests Only—or Prophets Also?

If the priestly orientation has dominated the professional identity of most physicians, the same is true of hospital chaplains. While the reasons for this are different, the broad picture has some similar lines. Recall that the priestly orientation has a strong ritual emphasis, a focus upon the individual, and a tendency to affirm the institution in which the priestly activity is carried out. The prophetic orientation, in contrast, emphasizes the ethical more than the ritualistic, has a more social than individual focus, and engages in constructive institutional critique. For more effective health care we need a redress in the balance, particularly a recovery of strength for the prophetic side that it might be held in creative tension with the priestly. This is beginning to occur among both chaplains and physicians, though unevenly and in different ways. Thus, our present situation invites considerable perplexity in professional identity and relationships. But at least some awareness of where we are and where we are going is important.

The troubled and hopeful years of the late 1950s and the decade of the '60s brought a resurgence of prophetic concern in the clergy as a whole. Nevertheless, for those in parish positions the focus remained rather heavily on the priestly side. One of the early and good sociological studies of churches in the racial crisis, Thomas F. Pettigrew's study of the Little Rock school integration, made a telling point: our religious institutions simply are not designed to support and reward prophets. The churches' institutional reward systems clearly accent the priestly functions —the performance of ritual activity, the care of the individual, and the upbuilding of the institution along those lines understood and affirmed by the majority of members.[1]

The same has been true, it appears, in hospital chaplaincy. In his recent book *Toward a Creative Chaplaincy,* Lawrence E. Holst describes that professional role in these words: "A *mediator,* a *mobilizer,* an *enabler*—that is the hospital chaplain today." [2] As a mediator, the chaplain is called to be a connecting link who stands between the patient and that person's own feelings about illness. The chaplain also stands between one patient and another, between the patient and family, and serves to connect these persons with the outside world and with God. As mobilizer, the chaplain helps to put into motion the healing resources within and between persons. As enabler, this minister facilitates and legitimates the growth and expression of faithfulness and concern toward the patient.

While that is a very good description of the priestly role of the chaplain, it is striking that this otherwise helpful description ends there. Virtually nothing is said about the prophetic dimensions of chaplaincy. Nothing is said about this minister's task in contributing to ethical discussions about the removal of heroic supports from the terminally ill patient; or the chaplain's task in stimulating from within the hospital some fresh thinking about our health care delivery system; or the chaplain's responsibility as a Socratic gadfly to the entire medical staff concerning the style of patient care; or the ministry of representing the hospital to its surrounding community with its own particular health needs, and representing that community to the hospital. On issues such as these there is silence.

Perhaps we ought not be surprised. A recent president of the College of Chaplains noted that not many years ago the institutional chaplaincy was conceived by both laypeople and clergy to be "a vocational spot for a minister who had given his best to some parish situation and now, in retirement, was wanting to continue to be active in ministry. Thus, the hospital was a good place for him to be situated."[3] Thankfully, this is no longer true. The chaplain has emerged as a professional among professionals. In the last quarter century the hospital chaplaincy has drawn on many disciplines, from psychology and psychiatry, from social work and education, from the health sciences and theology, to shape its self-image and equip its members for their tasks. The clinical pastoral education (C.P.E.) movement has developed national procedures and professional standards. The College of Chaplains has drawn together persons of varied ministries and has given them a professional identity and a professional home. Nevertheless, it seems fair to say that this first historical period of hospital chaplaincy has seen the dominance of the priestly mode of ministry.

Several years ago the late Robert A. Lambourne, an English psychiatrist-theologian, wrote a critique of the clinical pastoral training movement in America and its preparation of hospital chaplaincy.[4] It had become enamored, he claimed, by a psychological pietism. An "unconscious tribalism" had developed in which chaplains had taken their working models from the psychotherapists and developed a narrowness of viewpoint. Concentrating upon counseling, they had rarely given attention to the medical structures in which they were working. Concentrating on affirming the individual and nourishing his or her growth, they had separated love from justice. Focusing upon the individual, they had largely excluded the person's social context from the dialog—family members, place of work, neighborhood, or wider community. Using the psychotherapeutic model, hospital chaplains had developed a bourgeoisie mentality:

> ... the same ghetto situation in which a highly intelligent, privileged, and relatively affluent group developed a theory and practice of counseling in an isolated situation where problems of cultural relativity, stupidity, poverty, physical coercion, and so on could be ignored ... [with] the delusion that they were engaged in a universal process to which problems of justice and power were either secondary or irrelevant. Once again the theory and art of loving and acceptance were separated from the theory and art of justice and judgment.[5]

Lambourne's critique was directed toward a priestly class which had neglected the prophetic dimensions of ministry. In response, Seward Hiltner noted that Lambourne had not fully understood the American situation, though he had made some telling points:

> ... he does not recognize how deeply our "standard" programs of clinical pastoral education have been concerned with the poor, the underprivileged, the disinherited, the blacks and other minorities, and with those who are clearly not bourgois suburbanites. [However] I must honestly admit that, for far too long, our attempts to help these persons have not borne theoretical fruit in the form of a theology of justice emerging from clinical education.[6]

Yet there is mounting evidence that hospital chaplains are now moving to develop in theory as well as in practice the more prophetic dimensions of their calling. One piece of evidence comes from the professional literature. During recent years, the proceedings of the Annual Convention of the College of Chaplains have raised with consistent deliberateness the prophetic theme. In addition to the usual and legitimate concerns for ministering to particular needs of various types of hospital patients, one observes an impressive and increasing number of papers concerning the need for a more self-conscious ethical focus, the chaplain's role in community health, the chaplain's task in reassessing the whole health care delivery system, and the ministry of constructive critique of the hospital establishment. Interweaving throughout these concerns are persistent questions which chaplains themselves are raising about their own self-images, their ministerial roles, and their professional identities.

George Webber's comment is typical: "I assume this implies your prophetic role in the hospital is not simply to be a pastor to people but to be an *ombudsman*. I heard a college president ask Bill Coffin the other day, 'Chaplain Coffin, what is the job of a university chaplain these days?' He replied, 'to keep the president honest.' Well, can chaplains have that kind of relationship with the hospital, to keep it honest?" [7]

A similar accent on the prophetic comes from Carroll A. Wise, a well-known clinical educator. Writing about "The Chaplain of the Future," Wise notes that in light of the radical critiques which social analysts are now making of the health care system, chaplains will have to decide whether to be crusaders, supporters of the status quo, or creative and reconciling agents. "In short," says Wise, "the institutional ministry of the next few decades will be influenced greatly by the continued rise of scientific technocracy, by protests against this technocracy, and with this, close examination of the quality and costs of institutional care. The institutional chaplain cannot remain neutral and unconcerned with all of this. His task as a Christian pastor is that of being an agent of reconciliation, and he must learn how to do this." [8]

The Change Factors

While the movement in chaplaincy identity toward a greater balance between priestly and prophetic is still very much in process, it is worth singling out several contributing factors to this change. One of them, quite clearly, is the shifts which have taken place in theological education in the seminaries, changes which parallel those in medical education in the last two decades.

Traditional seminary curricula prior to the 1960s were arranged on a building block concept. During the first two years the student was required to give principal attention to several major theological fields—the foundation blocks upon which ministerial practice would later be laid. The seminarian during this period was immersed in the study of the Old and New Testaments, of church history and historical theology, and of systematic or doctrinal theology. Only after these foundation blocks had been secured did the student, toward the end of his or her seminary career, confront the issues of contemporary ministry and contemporary society.

Early in the decade of the sixties, however, a significant shift began to occur. Students were confronted at the very beginning of their professional education with the task of ministering and of doing theology in a rapidly-changing contemporary scene. Seminarians were placed for their required field work not only in parishes as youth group leaders but just as frequently in social agencies, drug rehabilitation centers, and community change organizations. One result was of pedagogical importance: students were immediately drawn into the contemporary relevance of theology and ministry, and, sensing that, they were motivated to dig back into the historical resources of the faith with more purposeful and livelier questions.

Another result, however, was that the very form of the questions tended to change. Instead of learning "Christian answers" to be applied to any and all situations, seminarians were pushed to discover what questions people were really asking in this time and place, what problems they were facing, what issues engaged them. And in light of those questions, the content of Christian ministry and theology could take meaningful shape—reflecting the Christian conviction of the perennial truth of the gospel and also the conviction that the gospel speaks in new forms and in new ways according to the needs of changing situations. And the situations in the 1960s and early 1970s reflected social unrest, national confusion, and radical questioning of established institutional patterns. Hence, the prophetic dimension of ministry re-emerged with considerable emphasis, and the hospital chaplain—whether actually in training during this period or on the job—felt and appropriated its impact.

During those same years a shift in clinical pastoral education also began to occur. It stemmed largely from two sources: the impact of urban ministry training and the impact of the new discipline of biomedical ethics. In surveying the American scene in 1968, Lambourne had observed a growing split between those who were teaching practical theology through counseling and clinical care and those who were teaching it through field work in depressed urban situations. The former leaned heavily upon psychology, the latter upon sociology. The former taught inter-personal sensitivity through immersion in the psycho-dynamics of the small group process, while the latter taught analysis and social change methods through selected exposure to cultural shock.[9] Lambourne's predictions, however, did not occur. The split did not grow between these groups; in fact, they influenced and cross-fertilized each other. Hospital-based programs began to take more seriously the neighborhoods of which they were part, and their students were found in free clinics as well as on the hospital wards. If the urban training centers helped clinical pastoral education to become more prophetically and socially aware, they were also helped by the clinicians to become more pastorally sensitive.

The emerging discipline of biomedical ethics also brought prophetic dimensions increasingly into the chaplain's role. The task of hospital chaplains of several decades ago was quite clearly defined: to minister to the religious needs of patients. Gradually a twofold expansion occurred in that definition. Chaplains began to see their ministry as one directed not only to patients but also to hospital staff members and to the institution as a whole; indeed, often their most effective impact upon patients was through other staff persons. In addition, the notion of "religious needs" underwent expansion. Certainly, the needs for prayer and liturgy, for comfort and counsel remained. But increasingly chaplains perceived that the ethical decisions which affected countless patients—decisions about heroic supports, about the allocation of scarce resources, about the experimentation conducted in hospitals, about the rights of patients and families—were also part of their ministry and laid claims upon their time and skills.

Biomedical ethics as a discipline has emerged only since the late 1960s. A core of professionals began to devote major time to this ethical area. Independent institutes for this purpose were established—notably the Institute of Society, Ethics and the Life Sciences at Hastings-on-Hudson, New York, and The Kennedy Institute for the Study of Bioethics and Human Reproduction in Washington, D.C. Periodicals specifically oriented to biomedical ethics emerged for the first time. And hospital chaplains, appropriately, were not untouched.

Interestingly enough, the present uncertainty in the definition of biomedical ethics as a field reflects the same problem in the hospital chaplain's self-definition. Roy Branson has labeled the ethical problem: workers in this field are not united in their answers to the question, "whether there should be an ethics *in* or *of* biomedicine." [10] Those who opt for the former tend to see biomedical ethics as an interdisciplinary *consulting* profession. Its basic task is to aid the physician in that professional's own decisions concerning what should be done to or for patients. Those who opt for the latter and broader definition insist that biomedical ethics ought to be viewed as a legitimate and independent academic discipline which develops its own theory and raises its own questions. Its task is not simply to assist doctors in solving the problems which they raise about individual patients. Its task is also to press those issues and raise those questions which the physicians, by and large, have not yet sufficiently faced—such as how hospitals and other medical institutions are organized and how the medical professions are relating to the real needs of society.

Thus, the chaplain-as-ethicist faces this question: Is the chaplain's role fundamentally a consulting role, dealing with only those issues which the doctors themselves raise? Or is the chaplain's ministry as ethical reflector more broadly conceived so that he or she operates collegially with physicians but also somewhat independently of them, raising up for public discourse any and every issue appropriate to the hospital's task in caring for human health? Prophetic dimensions of ministry are involved in both of these orientations, but the latter much more fully embraces the prophet's ethical task.

Theological Resources for Chaplaincy

As a specialized form of ministry, hospital chaplaincy draws on a wide and rich spectrum of theological resources for its tasks. Concerning the recovery of a more creative tension between the priestly and prophetic ministry in chaplaincy, however, consider just a few: [11]

First, since healing is one major sign of the redemptive activity of God, and since that redemptive activity is intended for all people, the chaplain is always called to care about justice in the health care system. To the extent that psychological individualism or a bourgeois tribalistic mentality exist, such orientations must be placed under the searching judgment of God's universal salvation. It is a salvation which is social *because* it is personal, caring about justice *because* it cares about love. The signs that Jesus is bearer of redemptive activity are clear enough: "the blind receive their sight, the lame walk, lepers are cleansed, and the deaf hear, the dead are raised up, the poor have good news preached to them" (Luke 7:22).

Second, since healing is fundamentally God's activity and not a human achievement, the human role is that of enabling and facilitating. Robert V. Moss says it well: "The church is called not to engage in healing, but to engage in a healing ministry." [12] The hospital chaplain shares in the New Testament perception of ministry—*diakonia*. "The word *diakonia* is rooted in a Greek word which means literally 'to wait tables'—to make it possible for people to eat. Thus a *diakonos* or minister is one who plays a subordinate role, is at hand, and assists." [13] But this does *not* mean that the chaplain plays the subordinate and assisting role to the physician. It means that both chaplain and physician, both nurse and social worker are always in subordinate and assisting roles to that healing process which they have no power to create but which they can facilitate. One certain way to lock the chaplains into a narrowly-conceived priestly role is to convince them that they are assistants to the physicians. One promising way of enlarging the role definitions of both professional groups is that they see themselves as collegial facilitators of a process whose source and power transcends all human agency.

Third, the patient needs to participate as fully as possible in his or her own healing process. Such typically was the case in Jesus' own healing ministry, and the implications for the chaplaincy are immense. In medicine (as in law) the practitioner's task traditionally has been to use a body of professional knowledge *on behalf of* the patient. In ministry (as in teaching) it has been otherwise. Here success has been measured, in part at least, by the minister's ability *to share* the body of knowledge, to enable the other person to understand and to become involved in what is going on. More recently, medicine and law, largely under the influence of liberation and human empowerment movements, are beginning to move away from highly paternalistic ways of relating to patients and clients. But this movement is only beginning.

Persisting Dilemmas and a Possible Image

The hospital chaplain, in struggling to develop and live out an appropriate professional identity, exists in two worlds. A minister by calling and profession, he or she also lives daily under the influence of the medical model. Further, the chaplain is subject to the continuing barrage of a variety of differing role expectations coming from patients, families, and hospital personnel. The persisting dilemmas are evident in the following comments, paraphrased from conversations with chaplains in major urban hospitals:

—I'm very conscious of the need to get in touch with the masculine side of my professional identity. The caring professions, of which ministry is a prime example, traditionally have accented the feminine. We are the nurturers and the supporters. These tasks are tremendously important, and I fully affirm them. But I also need to express those typically masculine traits in my work: initiating new approaches, challenging traditional styles of health care in this hospital. . . .

—I see an important part of my role as that of the educator. I need to ask the right questions of other people in the health care disciplines. I talk to a variety of groups in more formalized settings. The educational process with my parish clergy colleagues is important, too—assisting them to understand effective ways of ministry in the hospital setting. In a large hospital such as this, one chaplain, or even two or three, can't do the whole job. We have to enlist the ministries of numerous people. But many folks overlook, or don't really understand, this part of the chaplain's role. . . .

—For years I had to struggle to gain acceptance in this hospital for the kind of chaplaincy I believe important. And, to some extent, the struggle still goes on. Even after fifteen years here my presence is still viewed by some of the staff as one who does only the traditional priestly things, as one who represents only one particular denomination, and as one who is here only temporarily before going into "the real ministry," the parish. Gradually, I've been able to communicate a broader role definition to many of the staff, but with the usual staff mobility there are always some new faces on the wards, and so the interpretive process must go on. But it does take valuable time and energy. . . .

Surely, there are no simple answers. Yet, many are the chaplains—as indicated in the comments above—who daily work at the task of forging and communicating effective professional identities. They are embracing and affirming both the femininity and the masculinity of their humanness, knowing that ministry calls for both. Correlatively, they are expressing both the priestly and the prophetic, knowing that ministry demands both. And in doing so they are drawing upon the theological insights of Christian faith.

One image which might lift up some of the creative tensions important to the chaplain's unique situation is, on the face of it, an odd one: the circus clown. Heije Faber, a Dutch pastoral theologian, has suggested it.[14]

The comparison of chaplain to clown is in no way demeaning or trivial. Quite the contrary. The clown is indispensable to the circus. Without this figure, the circus is reduced to a string of individual acts. With the clown, it develops a certain meaning and coherence otherwise unattainable. Consider why this is so:

First, the clown both belongs to the team and yet has a different function from the others. The others all have something in common—the trapeze artists and the daredevils, the liontamers and the acrobats all rely upon skill and courage. But the clown seems to deviate from this norm. Likewise, the hospital chaplain frequently discovers that the medical staff, even when they try to understand, find it difficult to grasp the nature of the chaplaincy. For the clown, the public is less an object of the performer's prowess than it is people with whom the clown develops a "boundary situation" identification. So with the chaplain who seems not so much to exhibit marvelous skills which the patient wants to see, but rather identifies with patient and family in the boundary edges of their existence—in setbacks, in sorrow, in the seemingly absurd.

Faber suggests a second distinction: the clown appears to be the amateur in the midst of experts. When other performers do their great feats, the clown's skills seem pitiable by comparison. So also in the hospital. Within those walls are taking place amazing feats of medical science, and the experts of numerous medical fields all contribute to those wonders. On closer inspection, however, we realize that the effective chaplain must also be highly skilled and perceptive. But this is a different range of skills and understandings.

I believe that these first two facts of clowning accent the chaplain's priestly tasks. Here the clown represents the paradox of the divine foolishness—finding wisdom in foolishness and strength in weakness. So also the chaplain, through identification with patient, family, and staff, through sharing his or her own humanity, opens up others to more of their own humanity and mortality —their littleness but, strangely enough, also their greatness. That is authentically priestly work.

There is another essential facet to the clown which is, I believe, more prophetic. Here the clown is the court jester.[15] Here is the one, much more than simply joker, who perceptively punctures balloons. The jester pricks all pretensions, whether in institutional policies or in individuals, reminding us of our common humanity. The jester has the freedom to lift up new courses of action: "My lord, have you never thought of . . . ?"

Chaplains as jesters do not, I strongly suspect, have an easy time of it. They draw their paychecks from hospitals dominated by doctors and, as Thomas A. Harris says, "In the clubhouse of the doctor the chaplain has his locker and he doesn't want to lose his membership."[16] This minister knows of changes which ought to be made in our health care delivery system, but changes are always difficult and often painful to make. The chaplain knows that decisions about life and death matters involving patients ought to be made communally and not unilaterally, but it is sometimes risky to assert oneself. Very probably, not many court jesters lived to ripe old retirement ages. Undoubtedly many lost their pointed caps and bells (and maybe their heads) prematurely. But, difficult as their role was, that kind of clowning was necessary in the royal environs. Given the nature of the contemporary hospital, it is also necessary there.

Whether the image of the clown is useful in drawing together the roles of priest and prophet, the reader must decide. In any event, it is instructive to remember that there is a long history in our faith, reflected in its art and literature, of perceiving Christ himself as God's clown. What shall we say to that? "On with the show"?

4

The
Personal Needs
of Patients

In Judeo-Christian history "salvation" and "health" originally were very closely related. It is true in most of the Old and New Testaments. As the history of the church unfolded in early centuries, in spite of a continuing concern for some forms of healing, salvation and health began to be sundered in common thought. Salvation soon was thought to deal only with the person's spirit, and had little if anything to do with his or her body.[1]

Theology, even today when we are becoming more aware of the psychosomatic unity of the person, has dealt little with the *physiology* of alienation and grace. Our notions of a "graceful body" and a "disgraceful body" are superficial ones, having to do only with bodily shapes and movements which we find esthetically appealing. The state of theology on this matter signals the state of most Christian thought—we still are plagued by this dualism, even though we are increasingly aware that it does not do justice to the divinely-given unity of the person nor to an adequate theology of health and healing.[2]

But if the church tended to accent spirit, medicine did not escape this dualism; it simply reversed the accent. When medicine declined as art and rose as science, a mechanistic and materialistic understanding of the person developed. If the patient was not simply a fascinating machine in need of repairs, at least that patient was often thought of more as a case than as a person. It still persists whenever hospital personnel refer to "that appendectomy in 821" or "that hernia in 414," forgetting that we are not dealing fundamentally with an appendectomy but with Janice Black, not essentially with a hernia but with Charles White.

Two other biblical insights are of paramount significance in dealing with the patient as a person.[3] One is that the person in need of healing must participate actively in the healing process and not remain—or be forced to remain—passive. It is typical of Jesus' healing ministry that the great majority of persons who were aided by him were helped because they actively participated both through desire and through faith. Indeed, Mark makes a very sad comment, saying that Jesus could not work many miracles of healing in one community because of the people's lack of faith (Mark 6:5). So also in modern medicine, healing is not simply a bio-mechanical process which is applied to a patient; it is a restorative process in which the person's participation is crucial.

The other insight follows. We are not isolated individuals but persons-in-community, and the community should participate in the healing process as well as doctor, nurse, and patient. Again the pattern appears in Jesus' healing. The paralytic can be healed because of the faith of the four friends (Mark 2:5), and the epileptic boy's healing is mediated significantly through his father's faith (Mark 9:24). There is a healing community which extends beyond the immediate patient and medical personnel to include family, close friends, and in some important respects even the wider society.

Underneath these important assumptions about the unity of the person and the individual's and community's participation in the healing process lies a fundamental truth: the importance of *caring*.[4] In clinics and hospitals, in nursing homes and other health and welfare institutions, we are concerned about *curing* certain conditions. But if our attempts to cure are not to sunder the person once again, we need to be clear that our principal vocation or calling is to care. Curing is important and possible in many cases. Caring is fundamental and possible in every case.

And what does caring mean? While the question deserves volumes, at least we can say this. Caring is much different from sentimental compassion. Caring is an active attitude which genuinely conveys to the other person that he or she does really matter. It is different from wanting to care *for* another in the sense of making that person dependent on us. Rather, it involves a profound respect for the otherness of the other. It is grounded in the sense of uniqueness and worth which, by the grace of God, the other has. Caring is different from imposing my own sense of direction on the other; it involves commitment to the other person's own growth as a person, no matter what that person's age may be. Caring thus requires trusting the other's capacity for growth. Caring requires humility—a continuous learning about the other, an openness to the novelty of each new situation in which a mechanical application of the rules may not suffice. Caring requires hope in the possibilities which the future can yet bring. Indeed, the language and shape of caring are the language and shape of love. Yet, recognizing how the word "love" in popular use becomes sloppy in content, we might come at it freshly if we think of our vocation to *care*.

The Tasks of Human Growth

To care about patients is to care about persons who, regardless of their age, have certain basic needs for human growth. Erik H. Erikson, one of the justly-renowned psychologists of our time, has given us a picture of the eight stages of human life.[5] These are stages in the sense that each individual goes through different periods in life when a particular personal capacity needs to be developed. In another sense, however, we never leave any of these stages behind. Though their tasks are crucial at particular times of our lives, these various capacities must be *confirmed* and *reaffirmed* throughout our lives. Nowhere is this more important than in relating to persons who are ill. Here are Erikson's stages:

First, in early infancy, it is crucial that the child develop a sense of *basic trust over against a basic mistrust*. This comes with the infant's relation to significant adults, primarily the parents, and particularly the mother or the mother substitute. The amount of trust derived from early infant experience does not seem to depend on quantitative amounts of love or food given, so much as the quality of the relationship with the baby. When in later life mistrust prevails over basic trust, there are tendencies toward habitual depression or even schizophrenic states.

Second, during the second and third years of childhood the person must develop a sense of *autonomy over against shame and doubt*. Surrounded in his or her earliest years by a trusting environment, the child will not be jeopardized by the almost violent wish to make choices. If the nurturing environment encourages these choices it will also encourage a healthy autonomy. A sense of self-control without loss of self-esteem will emerge. But if the child's attempts to choose are met with ruthless control and constant shaming by adults, the child will develop a sense that its own demands and its own body are evil and dirty, a sense of doubt in its own ability for self-expression.

Third, is the stage of *initiative versus guilt*. Somewhere in the ages of three and four there is a new and vigorous unfolding of the child wherein he or she becomes more activating and energetically initiating. If the adult figures in the child's life can welcome this with gentle guidance and with little threat to themselves, a healthy initiative develops. If, on the other hand, the child's initiatives are met with persistent moralistic surveillance and prohibition, a syndrome of guilt develops, which later in life often emerges as a pattern of self-righteous intolerance.

Fourth, *industry versus inferiority* is the next task. In the years between pre-school age and puberty, the child learns to produce with skills and tools. Encouraged with appropriate instruction and inspiration, the child senses developing competence, but discouraged the child may consider himself or herself doomed to mediocrity and inadequacy.

Fifth, in adolescence comes the stage for developing *identity versus role confusion*. Here is a crucial stage, building on all that has gone before. Against the threat of confusion and diffusion—

too many selves to know the one true self—the adolescent's task is the development of a confident and comfortable sense of who he or she is.

Sixth, *intimacy verses isolation.* The young adult, emerging from the insistent search for identity, is now willing and eager to fuse his or her identity with that of others, ready to commit the self to relationships and stand by those commitments. But frustrated by the threat of intimacy, the person recedes into protective isolation.

Seventh, adulthood brings with it the task of *generativity versus stagnation.* Generativity is the concern for guiding the next generation, whether through parenting or other forms of productivity and creativity. Without generativity there is stagnation.

Eighth and last is the stage of maturity and old age: *ego integrity versus despair.* Here in old age, the healthy individual embraces his or her own life and accepts it as something which is and was and had to be. The lack of ego integration is signified by the fear of death—the feeling that time is now too short to start life over again, the disgust that life is not what it should have been and hence death must be warded off at all costs.

These, then, according to Erikson, are the basic psychological needs of persons: a sense of basic trust, autonomy, initiative, the capacity for industry, the secure sense of identity, the capacity for intimacy with others, generativity, and, in the later years of life, a sense of ego integrity. But remember: these are not simply stages through which a person passes and leaves behind. These are lifelong tasks, even though their development may come principally during a certain period. Also Erikson would have us remember this: the community of significant others who surround any person is crucial in helping him or her to reffirm these various capacities, abilities, and self-understandings.

An Illustration: Terminal Illness

The workings of these theological and psychological assumptions can be seen more clearly, perhaps, if we consider particular situations and needs in which patients find themselves. Terminal illness often presents a dramatic illustration. The following case is a factual one.[6]

Adolph Larson was an 83-year-old farmer with cancer of the prostate. Prostate surgery removed a portion of the cancer, and abdominal surgery relieved a kidney obstruction. Mr. Larson was moved to a nursing home, where he had now been for six weeks, lying in bed depressed, withdrawn, and with little interest in life. Here was a proud and independent man who had never been inside a hospital until six months ago when he developed prostate cancer.

Mr. Larson's daughter was angry about his deteriorating condition. She was not ready for him to die and wanted the doctor to instill in him the will to live. Hoping for better care, she changed his physician to a younger man who first spent considerable time talking with the patient, trying to understand him. Then the new doctor liberalized his strict diet, encouraged the use of colorful pajamas, radio, TV, and the regular wheeling of Mr. Larson onto the patio. The doctor had discovered that the patient's loss of control over his situation, including his bladder and bowels, was a source of deep shame and depression.

After some days of recovery of his spirits, Mr. Larson suddenly refused to eat, claiming, "Life is all over for me. . . . I want to end it all." After an initial attempt to cheer him up and to argue with him about his future, the doctor realized that he was not so much arguing with the patient as with himself and his own fears of dying. A few minutes later, the physician changed his course. "Do you feel this is the right time? Is your family prepared? How do you feel about dying?" Now Mr. Larson responded more freely. He was not afraid to die so much as he abhorred his increasing weakness, his having to lie in his own feces until an aide came to clean him up. This spirited, independent man was determined to do what he wanted, and would refuse food and water, accepting only pain medication if he became too uncomfortable. The doctor warned him that it might take him two weeks to die without fluids, but Mr. Larson insisted that he was ready to proceed.

He died fifteen days later, the doctor having visited him regularly without interfering in his wishes. Mr. Larson's daughter accepted his death with normal grief but with surprising calm.

In the language of medical ethics, this would be a case of voluntary indirect or passive euthanasia. The patient voluntarily chose to end his life by refusing or withdrawing from those things which would have prolonged his existence. My purpose at this point is not to debate whether or not Mr. Larson's decision was morally legitimate and Christianly defensible. I am assuming that it was. I am assuming that his voluntary passive euthanasia was ethically different from suicide. It was a decision made in a situation of terminal illness with motives, intentions, and consequences significantly different from those we think of as suicidal. What concerns us here is the manner in which the basic psychological needs and tasks of the life cycle are all present and expressed in Mr. Larson's case—and given less understanding staff persons these needs could have been thwarted and denied.

Consider the needs for trust, autonomy, and initiative. Mr. Larson needed to continue to trust himself, to experience himself as a trustworthy and worthwhile person. Given the nature of his whole life as one of rugged independence and self-control, he felt keenly the loss of his autonomy and his initiative in his final illness. His body had become uncooperative and degrading. His incontinence disgusted him. His desire for dignity and independence was as fierce as ever. But he was thrust into depression, mingling of shame and doubt and guilt, by his situation.

Mr. Larson still needed to maintain his strong sense of identity—his secure notion of who he had been and who he now was. Having been a generative, productive man, he feared the ultimate stagnation of his seemingly endless terminal illness. In his maturity and old age, he apparently had achieved a sense of ego integrity. He looked back without regret upon his life. He looked back, in fact, with a sense of due pride.

Through all of this experience in his final illness, the patient showed his need for intimacy. His withdrawing into protective isolation came only at those points wherein the significant others —his daughter, his doctor, the staff members—did not take his intimacy needs seriously. He needed to share with them exactly what he was feeling and why, and when they responded with false and evading cheeriness they only proved to him that they were rejecting who and what he really was now. When intimacy needs are repeatedly rebuffed, protective isolation seems the only recourse. The turning point came when the young doctor realized that his own attempts to argue with Mr. Larson about the future, to console him, to cheer him up, were mainly reflections of the doctor's own personal needs. It was the doctor who had the greater fear of dying. It was the doctor who did not want to "fail." It was the doctor who feared that he might look foolish to the nursing staff, having begun an aggressive rehabilitation program and apparently having misjudged his patient's will to live. But when he turned the corner, was able to set his own fears aside, and was able to meet Mr. Larson on the patient's own grounds, intimacy was reestablished.

The basic stages of the life cycle never leave us. Even in the last days of conscious life Mr. Larson exhibited his need for basic trust and autonomy, for initiative and industry, for a continuing sense of personal identity and intimacy, for generativity and ego integrity. Is it really any different for anyone in any of our health care institutions? And the interconnection of all these needs is striking. They are interconnected within the individual. But how the person is able to satisfy these needs depends so much on the responsiveness of those around him or her. Erikson sums it all up by showing that the first and last stages of life come together in a completed circle: "It seems possible to further paraphrase the relation of adult integrity and infantile trust by saying that healthy children will not fear life if their elders have integrity enough not to fear death." [7]

An Illustration: Sexuality

Though Freud can be debated in some other respects, surely he was right in labeling death and sex as very basic human problems. We can appropriately turn to sexuality for a second illustration of meeting the patient as a person.

For a variety of reasons we tend to "de-sex" persons in our health care institutions. Many of us would be more comfortable if patients simply were not sexual beings. Undoubtedly, some of these attitudes are rooted in our ignorance of sexual needs of persons in every stage of life, both in illness and in health. Some of our attitudes perhaps come from inherited religious and cultural beliefs about sexuality (see Chapter Five). And some of our discomfort may well express our own sin—the propensity to take ourselves as the norm by which all others should be judged, and hence to assume that those who are significantly different from us have no right to be as sexual as we are. In any event, consider three types of situations in which the sexual needs of patients frequently are poorly understood by the helping professionals who surround them.

The first illustration is the couple, one of whom has been diagnosed as having a terminal disease. This person still may have months to live, perhaps much of this time at home. And this person's sexual needs and anxieties during this period may be particularly great, but the professional typically treats this area with disconcerting silence. Such silence in itself may unnecessarily hasten the individual's loss of genital capacities simply because the patient has not received the needed affirmation and permission to continue as a sexual being. Another problem may arise from the partner's conflicting sexual needs and an absence of communication about them. For example, the healthy spouse is in the midst of anticipatory grief and is preparing for death's severing of the relationship. This partner may begin to withdraw from sexual expression, for sex seems too painfully a symbol of an ongoing and life-giving relationship. At this precise time, however, the ill partner may feel the need for, and have the physical capacity for, increased sexual activity. To the patient, increased sexual intimacy would counter death anxieties and express his or her profound investment in maintaining a vital couple relationship throughout the remaining time. Such distressing situations arise, but because physicians and pastors too readily assume that the terminally ill have ceased to be sexual persons, little help is offered. And when help is sought, the professional may not be prepared to give it.[8]

When the terminal patient is hospitalized, intimate sexual expressions with the spouse are usually impossible. The hospital is not set up to accommodate this need, however much the patient may benefit from it. In her autobiographical account of her slow cancer death, JoAnn Kelley Smith spoke to the point: "One of my strongest feelings about the hospital environment is that there should be two or three rooms equipped with double beds for conjugal visits. . . . I believe it should be possible for a husband or wife to stay with his or her mate, even if it is just overnight and if the patient doesn't need a lot of nursing care, particularly if it's a terminal disease."[9]

A second illustration concerns the patient in a nursing home, youth home, hospital, or mental institution, for whom genital expression in a committed relationship is impossible. Yet, many such persons, like most of the rest of us, have genital needs. Perhaps it is time that medical and religious professionals rethought the issue of masturbation. Even today the word "masturbation" seems to have an unsavory, unhealthful connotation. Medically, however, we need to know that there is no physiological harm whatever in such sexual self-release. We need to realize, also, why masturbation was viewed negatively by our religious ancestors—for reasons inapplicable today. It did not produce children (who were needed in an early and underpopulated society); and in males the practice was believed to be the deliberate destruction of human life (since in a patriarchal, pre-scientific society the male semen alone was thought to carry life). Psychologically, we need to realize that sexual self-stimulation need not be a sign of emotional maladjustment. Dr. David Cole Gordon laments the branding of all masturbation as arrested development or relational immaturity: "An activity which should be benign, if not beneficial, has become a source of much human suffering and anguish." [10]

All of us have deep needs to feel that our bodies are good and trustworthy. We need to express our autonomy and self-acceptance. For some persons the sublimation of genital desire is compatible with the fulfillment of these personal needs. But for others, genital self-expression is not simply a release of physical tension but is also a personally affirming and unifying experience. Such may be the case for many patients in health institutions, persons without partners in those situations. If so, it may well be the grace of Christian and human caring to afford them the nonjudgmental understanding and the physical privacy which they need.

The third illustration of patients' sexual needs leaves the matter of genital expression and returns to sexuality in its broader sense. This is simply the need for physical closeness and human touching. Erik Erikson suggests this in his discussion of trust, intimacy, and generativity. Modern psychosomatic medicine frequently recognizes the healing possibilities of physical touch, and long ago the ancient church recognized that personal healing often came through the laying on of hands. If our embodiment and our sexuality in its broadest sense is intrinsic and not accidental to our capacity for human loving, then we must take seriously the human need for physical as well as emotional touching.

A remarkable motion picture, *Peege* depicts the Christmas visit of an affluent suburban family to the man's mother ("Peege") in a nursing home. In a series of flashbacks we see her earlier days as she romps delightfully with each of her young grandchildren. Birthday parties, and summers at Peege's cabin, and dancing with Peege, and her penchant for double-dip ice cream cones, and Peege staying up with them for the late horror movies—all these are the memories which come flooding back to the three grandsons, now young adults. But today Peege seems a shadow of her former self; blind, bound to a wheelchair, unsmiling, communicating with only an occasional single word. The pain of the situation unfolds as the artificial cheeriness of the family's conversation grows increasingly more forced. They are saddened and perhaps even repulsed by her condition—her racking cough, her drooling, her unexpressive head limp to one side, the catheter tube visible at her leg. Yet their contrived conversation goes on— about Christmas decorations she cannot see, about people she does not know, about presents which have no interest for her.

But nobody gets physically close to her. No one touches her. The strained pleasantries of goodbyes are said, and the family leaves for their car. That is, all except the eldest, college-age son, who stays behind, making some excuse to the others. It is he who then comes close to her, puts his arm around her shoulders, his own cheek touching hers. And he talks. But this is a different conversation. It is about intimate memories they both recall. It is about Peege's own feelings. Where in the earlier moments with the whole family present there had been no real touching of life with life, now there was touching both in body and in spirit. Peege responds with almost a whole sentence, and, most importantly, with a smile. In the car on the ride home, the rest of the family cannot understand why the eldest son stayed and kept them waiting. They can only talk about how pitiful Peege is these days, how she can't seem to feel anything anymore. And the conversation quickly turns to things more pleasant. But the son is quiet, for the others do not understand.

These are stories of human needs: needs for trust and autonomy, needs for initiative and industry, needs for identity and ego integrity, needs for generativity and intimacy. These are the claims on us to care about the whole person. We might again lay claim upon great symbols of our faith to get us freshly in touch with these things—and with resources for responding to patients as persons.

5

Bodies,
Sexuality,
and Personal Health

We are not disembodied spirits. Persons are embodied. As we observed in the previous chapter, our attitudes toward our bodies are highly significant in personal health. Furthermore, our attitudes toward our bodies are deeply affected by our feelings and beliefs about ourselves as sexual beings. Awareness of this fact is growing in the medical community. Consider the following:

• The dean of a midwestern medical school estimates that between 60 and 70 percent of those persons now appearing at clinics and doctors' offices have no organic basis for their ailments. Indeed, they are physically hurting, though the root of the illness is not in a virus but in the emotions. And a large percentage of these diseases are linked to anxieties broadly sexual in nature.

• In 1974 the World Health Organization convened a meeting in Geneva on Education and Treatment in Human Sexuality. This gathering of clinicians and medical educators from around the world agreed that "problems in human sexuality are more pervasive and more important to the well-being and health of individuals in many cultures than has previously been recognized, and that there are important relationships between sexual ignorance and misconceptions and diverse problems of health and the quality of life."[1] The World Health Organization subsequently endorsed the following definition of sexual health:

Sexual health is the integration of the somatic, emotional, intellectual, and social aspects of sexual being, in ways that are positively enriching and that enhance personality, communication, and love.[2]

• Dr. Daniel H. Labby, professor of medicine and psychiatry at the University of Oregon Medical School, writes:

During illness, the loss of a sense of intactness, especially as related to body image, can cause great anxiety about the capacity to function sexually; feelings of self-worth and attractiveness to others are threatened at a time when need for intimacy is greatest. . . . Illness can so powerfully block normal expressions of feeling that sexual acting out occurs, sometimes in grotesque and socially unacceptable forms, reminding us that our sexuality is a critical component of our expressive life, necessary to general well-being, and devastating in its loss.[3]

• Finally, Dr. Richard A. Chilgren, pediatrician and Director of the Program in Human Sexuality, University of Minnesota Medical School, observes the intimate connection between sexual health and religious attitudes:

From my perspective as a scientist and medical educator, sexual health is but one of a number of quite rapidly emerging health issues that are being resolved by combining the healing arts of the scientist/physician and the theologian/minister. A good deal of accurate scientific information regarding sexual physiology and behavior has recently become available. When this factual information is combined with a search for meaning, an examination of values, and a reaffirmation of principles, powerful mechanisms are created to interrupt the cycle of fear, ignorance, and misplaced guilt that is at the root of almost all sexual problems.[4]

These medical voices are compelling. Sexual health and the overall health of persons are profoundly interrelated. Because of this, and because in our society attitudes about our sexual embodiment have been profoundly affected for both good and ill by the Judeo-Christian heritage, a theological reassessment of human sexuality finds a fitting place among these essays on personhood in medical care.

Lady Bennerley, one of the minor characters in D. H. Lawrence's *Lady Chatterley's Lover,* has this to say about the subject: "So long as you can forget your body you are happy . . . And the moment you begin to be aware of your body, you are wretched. So, if civilization is any good, it has to help us forget our bodies, and then time passes happily without our knowing it." [5] Obviously, the writer used Lady Bennerley as his foil. Indeed, Lawrence went overboard in his attempt to restore belief in the goodness of our embodiment, for he finally attributed to sex the power of salvation. But most of us, particularly in the Christian community, are less in danger of making sex our savior than we are in danger of continuing to experience an unnecessary and sinful alienation from our sexuality. The double messages, commonly heard, betray our ambivalence: "Sex is beautiful—but don't tell the children about it." Or, "Sex is dirty—save it for someone you love."

With all due credit to Lady Bennerley, my concern is not with a healthy unconsciousness of the body (after all, digestion is better when you are not aware it is going on). My concern, rather, is with those elements of alienation and rejection of our bodies, which for a great many Christians contribute to a desexed, disembodied self in a desexed, disembodied world articulated by means of a desexed, disembodied theology.

I am using "sexuality" as a broad, inclusive term suggesting our physical embodiment, our sensuality, our awareness of being female and male, our sense of incompleteness without the other, our experience of desire for the other. I am using "sex" as a narrower term to refer to the genital expression of our embodiment and sexuality.[6] We are all sexual beings, and self-affirmation in this respect does not mean the constant search for orgasms. Indeed, many a celibate person is affirmatively and joyously sexual.

Alienation of Self from Body in Our Culture

What about the alienation we experience from our bodies? Many will contest this point, noting that if anything we have a sex-drenched culture. From X-rated theaters to Masters and Johnson with their ingenious measuring devices, we seem to be inundated with sex. With a penchant for alliteration, Harvey Cox rightly comments that we use sex for *compensation* (it is the experience of the earthy in a plastic, neon world), with *compulsion* (our society doesn't go half way about things), with a high concern for *competence* (how to perfect your techniques, in paperback for $1.95), and as an instrument of *communication* (we could get to know each other better, more quickly, if we had sex, don't you think?).[7] But this, as Rollo May persuasively argues, is not so much an affirmation of our sexuality as it is a flight from the passion of eros by way of the sensations of sex. Thus sex becomes a dehumanized technique, a performance, a new puritanism, a new commandment to seek more intense experiences.[8] Paradoxically, then, the compulsive sex-consciousness of our present society may be one important sign of our alienation from sexuality.

Another sign of alienation is the manner in which we tend to distance the "self" from the body—in emotions, in attitudes, and even in physical sensations. Members of the helping professions are by no means immune. Dr. James W. Maddock speaks to the point: "If a patient does muster the courage to discuss intimate sexual problems or concerns, is the physician able to deal with them? Ample evidence shows that a professional's own anxieties about sex often obstruct his or her ability to assist others with sexual problems, or perhaps can lead to reactions that compound the patient's problems."[9] The same generalization quite fairly can be made of the clergy, to whom an even larger percentage of persons with consciously sex-related problems first turn.

Alienation, separation, sin—by whatever name this reality is called, it is always triadic in character: separation within the self, from other created beings, and from the Creator. Thus far we have observed some evidences of the self's internal disembodiment. We distance the mind from the body and experience the body as object. Indeed, with hints of the ancient body-spirit dualism we seem to find it more "natural" to say "I *have* a body" than to say "I *am* a body," as if the real "I" were quite detachable and independent.

What of the separation from other creatures? It is surely present in the ways we distance our emotions and physical expression from our human interaction. Much of our lives is conducted with calculated disembodiment, with rigid formalities regulating those socially-permissible public contacts—the handshake, the elbow grip, the polite kiss—even though athletes may be granted a temporary reprieve following the crucial play or the winning game. After his move to the United States, Paul Tillich wondered "how we in America managed to preserve any spontaneity and vitality at all in the face of our radical repression of bodily feelings. But in Germany," he observed, "there is often present a lustiness and heartiness of emotion, as shown for example in Luther's enthusiastic familiarity with fornication and defecation." [10]

Separation from our creaturely companions involves the whole of nature. Is not the split between body and mind, between spiritual and sensual, reflected in the split between ourselves and the earth? Separated from the rhythms of our emotions, are we not also separated from the rhythms of nature? Only belatedly are we realizing that in the great game of creaturely life we human beings may well make history by controlling nature, but to our chagrin we shall discover that "nature bats last." [11]

And what of our separation from God? One wonders why Christianity seems to produce more atheists than any other of the world's major religions.[12] One wonders about the impact of neo-orthodoxy's emphasis (still with us) on the total transcendence of God, God's radical otherness. In spite of some notable exceptions, it seems true of typical Protestant theology since Barth that nature has been dissolved in history and creation dissolved in eschatology. Rosemary Reuther is correct in observing that the newer theology of hope (as seen in Moltmann and others) is a dramatic expression of the inability to deal with the category of creation, the roots of which difficulty may well go back to Augustine's sharp disjunction between nature and grace in his debates with Pelagius.[13]

The technical formulations of theologians (for good and for ill) *do* have an impact on the person in the street and in the pew. There is still a strong religious suspicion of the human body and its sensations.[14] Thus, not too many years ago, some theologians believed that God must be declared dead in order that we might come alive. And they were partly right, for truncated *notions* of God must surely die. Indeed, God is revealed in history; God is radically beyond and transcendent. But God is also and at the same time One who is radically immanent, infusing nature, expressing divinity through embodiment and sexuality, rejoicing in sensual love. And these latter dimensions of the experience of God may be somewhat foreign to great numbers of Christian people.

The History of Our Alienation from the Body

The history of our Christian disembodiment is too long and complex (and perhaps well-enough known) so that only a broad brush stroke picture is needed here. The story culminates in the horror against sexual embodiment so well expressed by Hjalmer Soderberg in his novel *Doctor Glas:*

> Even today I've hardly recovered from my astonishment. Why must the life of our species be preserved and our longing stilled by means of an organ we use several times a day as a drain for impurities; why couldn't it be done by means of some act composed of dignity and beauty . . . ? An action which could be carried out in church, before the eyes of all, just as well as in darkness and solitude? Or in a temple of roses, in the eyes of the sun, to the chanting of choirs and a dance of wedding guests? [15]

Shades of Marcion who simply could not bring himself to think of God as the author of "the disgusting paraphernalia of reproduction and of all the nauseating defilements of the human flesh"! Yes, Marcion was a heretic. But there were others. There was St. Bernard, to whom the person was "nothing else than fetid sperm, a sack of dung, the food of worms." There was Tertullian, for whom woman was "the gate of hell." There was Origen who believed that original creation was entirely spiritual and sexless. And St. Jerome could bring himself to justify marriage only because it produced offspring who were virgins.

But, surely, it is a one-sided caricature to leave it here. We know the strong Hebraic doctrine of creation and its affirmation of the goodness of sexuality and the body. We know of Jesus' own participation in this embodied, creation-affirming world view. We recall the struggle of both Israelites and early Christians to keep a monotheistic faith pure from fertility religions with their idolatries and temple prostitutions. We can understand some of the concessions to Greek body-spirit dualism in the quest to extend the Christian faith to the whole inhabited earth and to communicate with non-Jews in their own thought forms. We can appreciate the power behind Paul's eschatology even when it seemed to leave sexuality behind. We can understand St. Augustine's regrets over youthful sexual folly, as well as his flirtation with the Manichaeans. And we can even perhaps understand the rationalist mentality of the medieval era wherein orgasm was suspect, because it was precisely at the peak of sexual intercourse that human reason seemed to evaporate. Indeed, centuries later one of a different mind-set, Alfred Kinsey, experimentally verified this phenomenon, the intensity of erotic union. Having graduated from the gall wasp, Kinsey took his research into the bedroom and fired blank pistols in the same room without disturbing lovers who were at the brink.[16] Perhaps the medieval rationalists had grounds for their suspicions. If erotic love is this strong, how could God stay in the picture unless eros were in some sense denied?

There are, I believe, three common attitudes toward sex and sexuality in Christian thought today.[17] The medievalists typify one of them: control by reason and the will. After all, is it not our experience that we can more easily master other appetites than we can master the sexual? We can come to terms with our greed, we can repress or sublimate our aggression, but our sexual appetite seems to leap up at inconvenient moments, revealing to us our animal state, taking possession of us with forces we do not understand. Instead of being our own master, we at times seem to become our own monster.[18] So we seek to control our sexuality for higher purposes through reason and will. And self-control easily slips into bodily mortification, the death of the flesh.

Thus a second attitude emerges. To counter the stringency of "the Apollonian" some would exalt "the Dionysian" within us. It is perhaps the oldest attitude of all, but also perennially new. Sexuality is seen as that which has been artificially repressed. Hence, throw off the social masks, this group would say. Rediscover your inner forces and feelings and at the same time you will be reunited with a cosmic vitality. Such a psychoanalytically and religiously sophisticated advocate as Norman O. Brown speaks in this vein. "But the curious feature of this school, even of its Christian members, is that they do not seem to regard sexual love or acts as ever truly *personal*." [19]

Then there is a third attitude: sex is unimportant—it is simply "there." Here is the take-it-or-leave-it approach, the approach of detachment. Sexuality is there, but don't make too big a thing of it. Tom Driver of Union Seminary, who almost a decade ago pioneered the modern theological recovery of the sexuality of Jesus, represents this view.[20] Jesus demythologized sex, says Driver, showing it to be neither divine nor demonic. We can have freedom over our sexuality only if we can take it or leave it. Sexuality thus becomes almost inconsequential and laughable (like the child laughing at the frog in the garden). We must be able to laugh at sex or be humiliated by it, for it is an irrational, impersonal force that threatens to turn even the best of us into caricatures of ourselves.

There is something amiss in each of these three schools of thought. Dan Sullivan is convincing in his criticism. What unites persons of each of these seemingly widely-differing approaches is a common theme: "the unyielding determination to locate human sex somewhere—or anywhere—outside the human self, the authentic 'me,' that inner core of personhood which makes humanity distinctive. In this one crucial respect, there is no difference between the Christian Fathers' conviction that sex is a 'beast in the belly,' and Norman Brown's that it is 'Christ in me.' " [21]

Reconciliation: The Self and the Body

In Christian faith, alienation is never the last word. The Apostle Paul speaks with power about both alienation and reconciliation: "Wretched man that I am! Who will deliver me from this body of death?" (Romans 7:24). I make bold to alter his words at this point, trusting that this revision also may be consonant with the gospel: "Wretched person that I am! Who will deliver me from this *death of the body?* Thanks be to God through Jesus Christ our Lord!"

The central Christian claim is that we have experienced God's reconciling activity through Jesus Christ. And crucial to this claim is the announcement that the saving presence of God is incarnate, en-fleshed, in a real human person.

Somewhere in Paul Tillich's writings I recall his asking, what child of four of five years of age has not contemplated the basic ontological question: what does it mean to *be?* As I reflected on that and tried to dredge back through my murky childhood memories, for the life of me I couldn't recall having raised the basic ontological question at that age. But I recall having pondered what was to me an important childhood religious question: did Jesus have a penis? After considerable inner debate I concluded, with a sense of righteous relief, that he did not. (Though I remember conceding that angels might have sexual apparatus, though in heaven surely no one would have to go to the bathroom.) It was not until two decades later in seminary that I realized that at a tender age I had succumbed to the Docetic heresy in Christology.

The age-old and perennial Christological heresy is still the Docetic one: the ancient body-spirit dualism applied to Jesus, the conviction more-or-less held by countless Christians that Jesus Christ could not have been fully human, that God could not (or would not) have become radically enfleshed, and that in Jesus we see God but only in the "appearance" of human flesh. The record seems unfortunately clear—that the church historically for the most part has presented Jesus as sexless. "And that for most people today is about the most effective way of saying that he was not fully human," John A. T. Robinson rightly observes.[22] Indeed, even to raise the question of Jesus' sexuality might be thought by some to be in rather poor taste. The Victorian within us still winces at the thought that the Incarnation might be "a tale of the flesh."

But the scandal of the gospel has never shied away from offending the tastes of the righteous. Yet, until very recently it was dreadfully difficult to find serious theologians willing to wrestle openly and fully with the question of Jesus' sexuality. Driver, William Phipps, Robinson—there are a few exceptions. Yet more often it is the artists and writers who have raised the question— from D. H. Lawrence to Nikos Kazantzakis to the rock opera *Jesus Christ Superstar*. Somehow they have sensed that what is at stake in this question (as in every Christological issue) is the very meaning and experience of our human salvation.

Our salvation does, indeed, hinge upon "the humanity of God," to use Barth's fine phrase. That humanity is an unexpected scandal, and the issue of Jesus' sexuality is a good place for testing our commitment to that humanity. Indeed, a non-physical interpretation of the Virgin Birth story still leaves unresolved the manner of Jesus' conception, and some biblical scholars suspect the possibility of an irregular sexual union. In any event, this line of reasoning ought not be rejected out of hand because of inappropriateness or impropriety. At the very least it prompts us to see the Incarnation in a fresh and even more scandalous light, a view that is hardly out of character for a gospel which proclaims that the divine love is often a surprising affront to our "normal" pretensions of human righteousness.[23]

In addition, we might have to take a fresh look at the debates of Nicaea and Chalcedon.[24] A persistent worry was that any insistence on Jesus' full humanity would lead to a denial of his divinity. Hence, the fears of men like Athanasius and Cyril led them to insist that the Word *became man,* but did not come into *a man.* "And they were prevented from understanding that men like Theodore and Nestorius really were arguing (as we can now see) for a genuine and deeply *personal* union of God and man in Christ—however inadequate their vocabulary . . ."[25]

Robinson correctly sees that Bonhoeffer's question, "Who is Christ for us today?" is the corollary of another question which Bonhoeffer asked himself, "Who am I?" "The mystery of the Christ is primarily a matter of *recognition*—not, Can you believe this individual to be the Son of God?, but, Can you see the truth of your humanity given its definition and vindication in him?"[26] And, I would add, can you see the truth of your embodiment and your sexuality given its definition and vindication in Jesus Christ? Can we see Christ at the very center of our fleshly consciousness? The vindication of the fullness of our embodied humanity? For what is at stake is the meaning and experience of our salvation, our recovery of wholeness, our reconciliation with that from which we have become separated. What is in question (here the Nestorians were right) is whether or not it is possible, however partially we may yet experience it, that there be a genuine and deeply personal communion of God and ourselves. And in regard to our sexuality and embodiment the question is whether or not we shall continue in a vain attempt to be more spiritual than God.

Who will deliver me from this death of the body? Thanks be to God through Jesus Christ our Lord! Christ continues to manifest the redemptive presence in movements of human liberation, and in our time the women's movement is a particularly important bearer of that presence. Rosemary Reuther trenchantly speaks to the link between our inner alienation and the subjugation of women:

All the basic dualities—the alienation of the mind from the body; the alienation of the subjective self from the objective world; the subjective retreat of the individual, alienated from the social community; the domination or rejection of nature by spirit—these all have roots in the apocalyptic-Platonic religious heritage of classical Christianity. But the alienation of the masculine from the feminine is the primary sexual symbolism that sums up all these alienations. The psychic traits of intellectuality, transcendent spirit and autonomous will that were identified with the male left the woman with the contrary traits of bodiliness, sensuality and subjugation.[27]

We need not document here the tragic and almost infinitely complex results in injustice and dehumanization which have flowed from male sexism. Suffice it to say, Christ as expressed through the women's movement brings a word of health. In our society the alienation from the body is a particularly masculine experience. It is more typically the male who relieves anxiety about his sexuality with locker-room humor and who feels driven to compulsive sex because he is not at home with his embodiment. What we now are beginning to realize is that a masculinized God oppresses all of us. If within each woman there is the masculine dimension and within each man the feminine, only a sexually-inclusive God can heal our fragmentation.

The vision and experience of God as sexually-inclusive is basic to our reaffirmation of the body; to our rediscovery of the importance of touch; to our renewed experience of wonder, fantasy, play, and that which transcends the rational; to our rejection of a distorted phallic and thrusting type of masculinity which has so raped the earth and violated its people.[28]

Such concerns are not simply feminine concerns. They are intrinsically part of the agenda of humanness into which the humanity of God beckons us. And how is that invitation given and received? Christian tradition answers: by grace, the free and unmerited loving activity of God. And how is that grace experienced? Again, Christian tradition answers: in the experiences of justification and sanctification. The words are ancient ones and may require continual reinterpretation, but the realities to which they point are perennial. Justification points to God's radical acceptance of us as persons without requiring that first we establish our worthiness. Sanctification points to the inner experience of God's presence whereby we can realize transformation and growth toward our intended human personhood.

How does this all apply to our sexuality? Consider first the symbol of *justification*. For many persons a powerful translation of this reality is found in Paul Tillich's well-known sermon, "You Are Accepted":

> It strikes us when our disgust for our own being, our indifference, our weakness, our hostility, and our lack of direction and composure have become intolerable to us. It strikes us when, year after year, the longed-for perfection of life does not appear, when the old compulsions reign within us as they have for decades, when despair destroys all joy and courage. Sometimes at that moment a wave of light breaks into our darkness, and it is as though a voice were saying: "You are accepted. *You are accepted,* accepted by that which is greater than you, and the name of which you do not know. Do not ask for the name now; perhaps you will find it later. Do not try to do anything now; perhaps later you will do much. Do not seek for anything; do not perform anything; do not intend anything. *Simply accept the fact that you are accepted!*" If that happens to us, we experience grace.[29]

Those are powerful words for us, for they point to a Reality which we have experienced—at least in moments and at least in part. But when we have experienced that grace we know it to be real. Yet, sad to say, so frequently we forget that the word of acceptance is addressed to the total self and not to a disembodied personality. *You* are accepted, all of you! Your body, which you often reject, is accepted by that which is greater than you. You are accepted in your sexual feelings and in your yearnings. You are accepted in those moments of sexual fantasy which come unbidden and which both delight and disturb you. You are accepted in your masculinity and in your femininity, for each of you has elements of both. You are accepted in your heterosexuality and in your homosexuality, for each of you very likely has elements of both. Simply accept the fact that you are totally accepted.

Can you see the truth of your sexuality and your embodiment vindicated in Christ? He is no sexless, Docetic apparition, but the enfleshment of God in a human being. Can you also see that the gracious word of acceptance frequently comes through the hidden Christ, the Christ incognito? It may be in the ecstasy and playfulness of sexual communion with your beloved. It may be in such a simple act as the spontaneous hand placed on your arm by a friend, but in that moment you were aware of healing.

Justification by grace calls forth our response. Martin Luther was suspicious of speaking of human love for God. He preferred to talk of *faith* in God and love for the neighbor. Indeed, when Luther's sturdy hymns of faith are compared with the romanticized love hymns, the point becomes clear. Somehow, the pallid eroticism of "I come to the garden alone" doesn't hold up beside the sturdy faith expressed in "A mighty fortress is our God." And yet we may have unduly neglected the possibilities inherent in Jesus' invitation to *love* God (and not only to have faith in God). Furthermore, we may have unduly neglected the healthy erotic dimension of love for God.

The erotic and sensual qualities of our response to our acceptance need not be written off because we are offended by the banalities of the 19th century romantic hymns. Indeed, recall the sexual imagery employed in the Bible to depict our invited relationship with God. Here is the Apostle Paul (for all of his other suspicions of the sexual relationship) boldly calling the church "the bride of Christ," and the apostle was steeped in the Jewish tradition which held that an unconsummated marriage was no marriage at all. And here are Paul's prophetic predecessors, Ezekiel and Hosea, likening Israel to the bride of Yahweh. Listen to Hosea: "I will betroth you to myself forever, betroth you in lawful wedlock with unfailing devotion and love; I will betroth you to myself to have and to hold, and you shall know the Lord" (Hosea 2:19). "You shall *know* the Lord." When we recall that the verb "to know" also connoted sexual intimacy to these writers, when we remember that to the Hebrew "knowing" was found in a relationship at once deeply personal and affectional, with no sharp separation between love and sex, these statements jar the mind and the senses.

Especially in the Protestant tradition, we have written off this possibility too quickly. We are beginning to realize that Christian love defined exclusively as agape (self-giving) without the dimensions of desire and receiving, libido and eros, may well be an impoverished and impoverishing love. To be sure, agape transforms the libido and the erotic to release them from possessiveness and self-centeredness, but it transforms and does not annihilate these other dimensions of our loving. Again we are driven back to the sexuality of Jesus. Should it be shocking to us to think that Jesus, while to the best of our knowledge remaining celibate, was moved by eros and libido as well as by agape? It is hard to imagine a deeply human tenderness (which the Gospels portray as so characteristic of him) that is not in some significant ways fed by springs of passion. "The human alternative to sexual tenderness is not asexual tenderness, but sexual fear."[30]

We cannot disembody and desexualize ourselves without inner alienation. But much in our received religious heritage seems to tell us that eros and libido, desire and sensual passion, have no place in our relationship with God. Much in our religious ethos resists the notion that sexual love is related to the very Ground of our Being. Why so many atheists in Christian cultures? If God's transcendence swallows up and negates God's imminence, if God's agape destroys God's eros, then perhaps we understand why. But the liberating and gracious word of the gospel is otherwise. "I have come that you might have life and have it in all its fulness" (John 10:10). You are justified by grace. You are accepted, the fleshly, embodied "you."

You are justified, and you are *sanctified* by the grace of God in Jesus Christ. You are invited to accept your acceptance. And as we appropriate the meaning of our acceptance, there are implications for the transformation of our consciousness, for the transformation of our action, for the transformation of our very being. Such is the message of sanctification.

But too often sanctification, as commonly understood, takes on overtones of growth in a kind of holiness which is progressive disembodiment. A clever parody of this was posted on the door of a seminary dormitory room in which I was staying during a meeting a few years ago. The seminary was a Methodist school, and the student who regularly occupied that room obviously had been instructed in Wesley's eagerness for Christian perfection and sanctification. On the door was posted a graph bearing the title "Growth in Grace." It looked for all the world like a business chart in 1929. The sanctification-growth line moved progressively upward to a high peak, but then took a sharp and devastating downward plunge. One comment was penned in beside the crash: "Met Dorothy."

If, however, our growth enabled by our acceptance by the Cosmic Lover (to use Norman Pittenger's felicitous term) is not a progressive disembodiment but includes rather a fuller realization of our embodiment and sexuality, what might it look like? The psychologist Abraham Maslow, writing about love and sexuality in "self-actualizing people," furnishes some helpful clues. The subjects whom Maslow studied in this regard he says "were loved and were loving, and are loved and are loving." [31] Listen to some of his characterizations of their sexuality.

• Genital sex acts seem to be wholeheartedly enjoyed, enjoyed far beyond the possibility of the average person, and yet specific sex acts do not play any central role in the philosophy of life. "In self-actualizing people the orgasm is simultaneously more important and less important than in average people."

• The sex act itself may bring on mystical experiences on some occasions, and yet at other times may be experienced in a light-hearted and playful manner.

• There is "a healthy acceptance of the self and of others." These people are much freer than the average person to admit the fact of sexual attraction to others, but they are less driven to love affairs outside their marriages.

• They talk more freely and casually about sex than the average person. Their acceptance of the facts of life, together with a more intense, profound, and satisfying love commitment "seems to make it less *necessary* to seek for compensatory or neurotic sex affairs outside the marriage."

• They do not sharply differentiate the roles and personalities of the two sexes. "These people were all so certain of their maleness or femaleness that they did not mind taking on some of the cultural aspects of the opposite sex role."

• Their healthy love relationship is characterized by "fun, merriment, elation, feeling of well-being, gaiety."

• There is the affirmation of the other's individuality, an eagerness for the other's growth, a basic respect for the other's unique personality.

Maslow's picture may be one significant portrait of sexual sanctification—the personal growth which is possible when we know that we are, indeed, accepted. Though he is not using theological language, the psychologist is pointing to the conjunction of these two dimensions of reconciling grace, justification and sanctification: "I have suggested that self-actualizers can be defined as people who are no longer motivated by the needs for safety, belongingness, love, status, and self-respect because these needs *have already been satisfied*."

We have only begun to realize some of the ways in which sexual health—the integration of the bodily, emotional, intellectual, and social dimensions of one's sexuality into enriched personal identity and capacity for relatedness—is a major health issue. In its recent attempt to define sexual health, the World

Health Organization took an unprecedented step. For the first time a major health organization officially used the term "love" in its understanding of health. The medical and the theological dimensions of personhood no longer can be artificially separated. In both theory and practice this realization can have immense implications for patients and their families, for medical professionals and for clergy. After all, the physiology and psychology of our human embodiment, our sexuality, are intrinsic and not accidental to our capacity for human loving and fulfilled personhood.

The poignant account of a close friend and clergy colleague speaks to the issue. His mother was dying of cancer. Her body was clearly showing the ravages of the disease, and she was distressed by her altered appearance. On the one hand, she was resistant to the visits of those close to her because of her disfigurement. Yet, at the same time, her need for physical closeness and personal intimacy was great. Her son came to the hospital to visit, and as they talked he rubbed her back to relieve some of the pain. After a time, sensing her need for even greater closeness, he lay down on the hospital bed beside her and held her closely in his arms. In that position they talked for a long time that afternoon, sharing thoughts and feelings more deeply than ever before. Later that night she died.

If our embodied sexuality is intrinsic to our capacity for personal love, in Christian faith we believe that authentic human love takes its shape from divine love. And the story we tell about divine love is a story of incarnation, death, and resurrection. Again, Thornton Wilder in *Our Town* seems to sense something of the interconnections. It is the scene wherein Emily Gibbs, having died during childbirth, is allowed (through the miracle of the playwright) to turn back the clock a number of years, leave her grave on the hill above Grover's Corners, and return to her family for one day—her twelfth birthday.

Emily appears in the kitchen that morning, where her mother is busy fixing breakfast. "Oh, Mama, just look at me one minute as though you really saw me. Mama, fourteen years have gone by.

I'm dead. . . . But just for a moment now we're all together. . . . Let's look at one another." Mama, however, is too busy.

So goes the day. People are too busy to notice. Somehow they are not touching each other. Finally it is too much, and Emily cries out, "I can't go on. Oh! Oh. It goes so fast. We don't have time to look at one another. I didn't realize. So all that was going on and we never noticed. Take me back—up the hill—to my grave. But first: Wait! One more look. Good-by, good-by world. Good-by, Grover's Corners . . . Mama and Papa. Good-by to clock ticking . . . and Mama's sunflowers. And food and coffee. And new-ironed dresses and hot baths . . . and sleeping and waking up. Oh, earth, you're too wonderful for anybody to realize you. Do any human beings ever realize life while they live it?— every, every minute?" A moment later Emily finds her answer: "The saints and poets, maybe—they do some." [32]

Perhaps the divine passion of death and resurrection is not as foreign as we have sometimes believed to the meaning of our human sexuality. For in death and resurrection lies the meaning of incarnation. And in incarnation lies our hope and our possibility of reclaiming joyful embodiment—which is a basic dimension of human health.

6

A Case Study
in Personhood,
Decisions, and Death

The Questions

Hovering over every significant medical issue are two questions: what should be done in this case? and, who has the right to decide? Each of the questions has its own importance. Yet, they are different issues, and a considered answer only to one of them in a medical situation is insufficient. Though different, they are also obviously interrelated in practice, for the shape of a particular decision will be affected by the roles and relationships of those who make it and who have the power to carry it through.

The case which follows is one with which I am intimately acquainted. It is worth reporting not because it is highly unusual. In the end, its newsworthiness was only that of the usual obituary column. Rather, it is worth reporting because undoubtedly there are thousands of close parallels occurring at this very moment, because there will be many more in the years ahead, and because this case and those similar to it raise so many of the difficult but personally momentous questions surrounding current medical care.

The Case

John Gage was a handsome, dignified man of seventy-three when his first stroke occurred late in January. He died seven months later, still handsome in appearance but with the indignities suffered by those who have had progressive and massive brain damage; loss of control over limbs, bowels, and bladder; and loss of capacity for speech and rudimentary interpersonal relationships. While his physiological death occurred in August, the death of his personhood had occurred gradually but unmistakably far earlier.

Mr. Gage had maintained an active retirement, working part-time as an official for the city of Plainville, a midwestern community of 3500. Constantly aware of health problems in his later years, he had long coped with angina pectoris and diabetes, and was hospitalized with a heart attack six months before his first stroke. Aware of the possibility of being heroically maintained and his dying unduly prolonged, Mr. Gage, while still in relatively good health, had frequently expressed his resistance to such procedures. The experience of the protracted death of his own mother and the prolonged invalidism of his sister had firmed his convictions.

His first stroke in January left him with paralysis of the left side (he was left-handed) and loss of speech except for aphasic, automatic sounds. After two weeks of hospitalization he was moved to a nursing home in Bigtown, some forty-five miles distant from his home, where speech and physical therapy were available. Several weeks of therapy, however, produced no improvement. Mrs. Gage remained in Bigtown with him, spending most of each day at his side. The three adult children—Jane, Don, and Bruce—and their spouses made frequent visits, often remaining for some days with him.

During the first weeks in Bigtown, Mr. Gage still had some capacity for recognition and made frequent attempts to communicate. He clearly conveyed despair over his condition and disgust over his incontinence. His wife and three children gradually came to a clear agreement. If it became conclusive that the brain damage was irreversible and if further debilitation occurred, no heroic medical measures should be used for him. Keeping faith with their husband and father, and expressing their own

Christian values in this sad situation would mean their cooperation with his dying.

Mr. Gage's physician of some twenty years would not promise
to support the family's convictions. By her own values and training, Dr. Farber said, she was bound to support and prolong life
with the appropriate medical means. Death was the doctor's
enemy, and in each case she must bear the final responsibility for
the course of medical treatment. A plaque hanging over the regis-
tration desk in her clinic bore these words:

> Hold the physician in honor,
> For he is essential to you, and God it is who
>   established his profession.
> From God the doctor has his wisdom,
> Thus God's creative work continues without ceasing,
> He who is a sinner toward his Maker will be defiant
>   toward his doctor. (Sirach 1-15)

An insulin reaction occurred in mid-March, producing further
brain damage and additional loss of recognition and communication. Mrs. Gage and the three children were unified in their
desires: no resuscitation in case of heart failure, no intravenous
feeding, no antibiotics in case of pneumonia, and a preference
for the withdrawal of insulin. Dr. Farber remained firm in her
position. Reaction from the three registered nurses in the nursing
home was mixed: one expressed complete support of the family's
convictions; one was strongly and verbally opposed; and the
head nurse vascillated but insisted that she would always carry
out the doctor's orders.

Since the therapy in Bigtown had been to no avail, and since
an opening occurred in the intensive care section of Plainville's
main nursing home, Mr. Gage was transferred to his home town
in mid-April. There he was placed under the care of a different
physician, Dr. Blecker, who displayed at least some openness to
the family's convictions. Early in May, Mr. Gage experienced
another trauma, later diagnosed as an additional stroke. Following this, his powers of personal recognition appeared to cease and

physical responses became only automatic. While the new physician agreed to no resuscitation in case of heart failure, he could not agree to the withdrawal of the supportive heart and diabetes medications. Plainville nurses and aides gave excellent care, and the nursing home took rightful pride in its concern for both patients and families. Nevertheless, the administrator gave no indication of willingness to support the family's wishes even if the doctor should concur. Mr. Gage's minister visited him periodically but without entering into discussion with the family concerning their feelings.

For the next two months, Mr. Gage's condition was stable. He regularly was given digitalis and diuretics for his heart and insulin for his diabetes. He was fed by mouth and ate well. Though his responses to stimuli around him were only rudimentary and automatic, family members spent hours with him each day.

In mid-July Dr. Osborn, a staff neurologist from Eastern Hospital in Metropolis, phoned Jane Gage Williams and her husband. A personal friend, he was concerned about the situation and volunteered to fly to Plainville to give a consulting opinion. With the cooperation of Dr. Blecker, the consultation was arranged for a week hence. Dr. Osborn spent a day in Plainville, first doing a neurological examination, then consulting with nursing home staff and the local physician. His examination confirmed massive dementia: irreversible damage to the higher brain capacities. But, as Dr. Osborn noted, other organ systems appeared stable, and with the good physical care the patient was receiving he might possibly live in his present condition for a couple of years. His recommendation: concur with the family's expressed wishes, withdraw the insulin, and allow Mr. Gage to slip into coma and die a relatively peaceful death.

Dr. Blecker was cooperative in his response, indicating, however, that the feasibility of withdrawal would depend upon agreement from his fellow clinic physicians and the nursing home administrator. The latter, Mrs. Swan, was adamantly opposed. It was morally wrong, she declared, to make judgments about life's quality. The withdrawal of life-prolonging medication was an affront to God and would threaten the morale of the entire nursing home. Mrs. Gage and her daughter Jane pressed the issue, even to the point of requesting a meeting of the nursing home board to review the administrator's decision, but to no avail. By this time the Gages' minister and another of the Plainville clergy were aware of the issues with which the family was struggling. They indicated the desire to support the family and be interpreters of the issues.

By mid-July three options remained. One was for the Gage family to accept the situation as it existed at the Plainville nursing home: the continuance of medical supports and Mr. Gage's probable transfer to the local hospital for additional procedures should a dramatic change occur. The family continued to believe, however, that this would be further prolonging the dying process and not a prolonging of personal life.

The second possibility was to remove Mr. Gage from the nursing home, taking him home where the family would have control over his medications. This, however, seemed unworkable. While Dr. Blecker indicated his possible cooperation with this option, it appeared impossible in Plainville to find the 24-hour private nursing care which the patient would need.

The remaining option was selected by the family: the patient's transfer to Metropolis several hundred miles away, where he would enter Eastern Hospital as a patient of the neurologist, Dr. Osborn. There additional neurological tests would be administered and, if the earlier diagnosis of irreversible dementia were confirmed, supportive medications would be withdrawn at the time of Mr. Gage's transfer to a Metropolis nursing home.

Early in August, Jane Gage Williams accompanied her father on the flight of the air ambulance from Plainville to Metropolis. Mrs. Gage arrived by car the same day with other members of the family.

At Eastern Hospital extensive neurological testing confirmed the earlier diagnosis. Dr. Osborn had discussed the case with other members of the medical and nursing staff, who subsequently gave the family their full cooperation. The three hospital chaplains, also personally knowledgeable about the Gage case, made special efforts to be with the family in supportive and affirming ways. Two days later the patient was transferred to Elmbrook Nursing Home where Dr. Osborn and an internist colleague gave orders that the only medications be sedatives for pain. The doctors kept closely in touch with both patient and family. Within a day of his transfer to Elmbrook, John Gage died with family members at his bedside.

Two Questions about the Decision

Two particularly perplexing issues are involved in the decision which was made on behalf of Mr. Gage. First is the distinction between *withholding* supportive medical measures and *withdrawing* them. Second is the distinction between *ordinary* treatments and *heroic* or *extraordinary* therapies.

As to the first issue, the opinions of the medical personnel obviously were at variance. Mr. Gage's Bigtown physician, Dr. Farber, was committed to maintain and prolong life, a viewpoint fully shared by Mrs. Swan, administrator of the Plainville nursing home. With a resistance toward making any value judgments about the patient's quality of life, they were firmly set against withdrawing any medical therapies presently in use and, in addition, showed reluctance to approve the withholding of additional measures which might still be applied. Dr. Blecker early indicated his willingness to make the distinction. Yes, he said, he could justify withholding such heroic measures as resuscitation in the case of heart failure. Following Dr. Osborn's neurological consultation, Dr. Blecker moved one step further: he was willing to withdraw certain of the supportive medications then being given. His reluctance to commit himself to a course of complete withdrawal, he said, was due less to his personal convictions than to the necessity for cooperating with the nursing home administrator, respect for the convictions of his more conservative clinic colleagues, sensitivity to the attitudes and mores which he thought were prevalent in Plainville, and concern about possible legal difficulties. The third position—withdrawal as well as withholding of medical supports—was that of Dr. Osborn and the chaplains of Eastern Hospital, after each had become thoroughly familiar with the details of the situation.

What of the commitment to use all medical measures available regardless of the patient's quality of life?[1] This position finds little support from major religious bodies and theologians. Two decades ago Pope Pius XII declared that physicians had no absolute obligation to use extraordinary means in cases of terminal illness: "Normally one is held only to use ordinary means according to the circumstances of persons, places, times, and cultures, that is to say, means that do not involve any great burden for one's self or another."

More recently, the General Synod of the United Church of Christ expressed the same conviction, and in addition left open the possibility of withdrawing medical supports as well as withholding them. Its pronouncement urged that the needs of the whole person always be kept paramount. After warning about the temptations in terminal care toward biological idolatry, the Synod declared:

> The supreme value in our religious heritage is derived from God the giver of personal wholeness, freedom, integrity and dignity. When illness takes away those abilities we associate with full personhood, leaving one so impaired that what is most valuable and precious is gone, we may well feel that mere continuance of the body by machines or drugs is a violation of the person.[2]

In certain situations, then, it may not only be morally *permissable* to discontinue therapeutic supports, it may actually be morally *obligatory* to do so. Such was the conviction to which the Gage family came.

Several surveys of doctors' attitudes show that the majority make a practice of withdrawing therapeutic supports in some types of terminal cases. On December 4, 1973 this practice was finally endorsed by the House of Delegates of the American

Medical Association: "The cessation of the employment of extraordinary means to prolong the life of the body when there is irrefutable evidence that biological death is imminent is the decision of the patient and/or his immediate family. The advice and judgment of the physician should be freely available to the patient and/or his immediate family."

Yet, various factors cause some physicians to resist such cooperation with the dying process:

• a higher death fear among doctors than among comparable professional groups;

• the weight of tradition and training in a generally conservative profession;

• the fear of erosion of confidence in doctors by patients and the community;

• anxiety about possible malpractice suits or criminal indictments for homicide;

• and, of course, some doctors simply believe that every patient's death is a professional failure regardless of the circumstances which surround that dying.

Even the language becomes confused. In the treatises on medical ethics there is little unclarity, however. *Active* euthanasia (*positive* or *direct* euthanasia) is the intentional causing of a terminal patient's death by deliberately administering some relatively painless death-dealing process. *Passive* euthanasia (*negative* or *indirect*), on the other hand, is allowing the terminally ill individual to die because of his or her disease by withholding or withdrawing those medical therapies which promise no meaningful recovery. Nevertheless, some physicians and others use *active* euthanasia to refer also to the withdrawal of medical supports. The same people reserve the term *passive* euthanasia only for those instances in which an extraordinary or heroic medical process which might be used is withheld from use. It is an unfortunate, if understandable, confusion of terms.

Ethically, the matter hinges on the distinction between "acts of commission" and "acts of omission."[3] Active euthanasia is, indeed, an act of commission. As an active procedure to bring on death, it differs from passive euthanasia in its psychological effects, in its possible social effects, in its deliberateness. Most of the ethicists who would approve of active euthanasia in certain tragic and extreme situations would still insist on the important moral differences between the two forms, and would strongly prefer the indirect or passive form.

Passive euthanasia—either in its withholding or its withdrawing mode—is an act of omission. While there is no disagreement on this concerning withholding medical supports, the confusion comes at the point of *withdrawing* them. In order to withdraw or discontinue, someone has to *do* something—disconnect the respirator, stop the kidney machine, write an order for discontinuance of medication on the patient's record. And this action necessary to discontinue appears, to some at least, to be the commission of something more than an omission. Psychologically this may be understandable. But it hardly makes ethical sense. The ethically significant difference lies in the immediate cause of death. In active euthanasia though the patient is terminally ill the immediate cause of death is the action of another person— the injection of air into the veins, the giving of a lethal dose of morphine. In passive euthanasia the immediate cause of death is the patient's own disease; for considered moral reasons, the patient has been allowed to die of the disease without further medical interference.

Paul Ramsey has observed:

> . . . for the moralist, a decision to stop "extraordinary" life-sustaining treatments requires no greater and in fact the same moral warrant as a decision not to begin to use them. Again if I have understood the medical literature, a physician can make the decision not to institute such treatments with an easier conscience than he can make the decision to stop them once begun.[4]

This was true in the case of John Gage. Dr. Farber certainly but also Dr. Blecker indicated more willingness not to begin a treatment than to discontinue one. They were reflecting a rather common medical distinction.

On the other hand, Dr. Osborn was thinking more like a moralist than like a typical physician. (Interestingly enough, this physician was widely-read in the literature of medical ethics.) To him, to the hospital chaplains, and clearly to the Gage family, the act of withdrawing medications from John Gage was an omission, an act of cooperating with a dying man and mercifully refusing to prolong that dying further. It was a refusal to sacrifice the caring for this particular individual to a general principle of life's absolute sanctity regardless of its quality. In their judgment, there had come a time in this sad illness when it was the higher act of caring and the more adequate reflection of God's will to say: "Enough."

The second, related ethical issue hovering over the months of discussion of John Gage's situation was the distinction between *ordinary* medical supports and those considered *heroic* or *extraordinary*.[5] Traditionally, moral theologians have termed *ordinary* those medical treatments which offer reasonable hope of benefit to the patient and which do not involve excessive pain, expense, or major inconvenience. *Heroic* treatments, on the other hand, do not promise reasonable benefit and cannot be administered without excessive cost, pain, or considerable inconvenience. Physicians tend to think more pragmatically, perhaps, speaking of ordinary treatments as those which are medically established and customarily used in a given illness.

Granted, the terms are relative ones. They depend upon both time and place; they depend upon the state of medical science at the moment and what is available or obtainable where the patient is being treated.

Nevertheless, though the line between ordinary and heroic is sometimes fuzzy, these are important distinctions which medical professionals, ethicists, and persons involved with the care of the dying continue to use. They are useful because they give guidance as to what is responsible medical care in particular cases. The guiding principle usually holds that heroic treatments are optional and depend upon the patient's circumstances. In John Gage's case the question became this: given the amount of brain damage which had already occurred, were the digitalis, diuretics, and insulin to be considered ordinary treatments? Or were they extraordinary?

By some of the criteria, they were clearly ordinary. The medications were easily obtainable. They could be used without undue pain. They were relatively reasonable in expense. And, surely these medications are routinely used for such heart and diabetic conditions, for they promise the benefit of keeping these diseases under control.

The key question, however, was this: granted that these medications benefited certain of John Gage's *diseases,* did they promise reasonable benefit for *John Gage?* If pneumonia had occurred, what about antibiotics? Surely, their application would have given reasonable hope for benefit in regard to the pneumonia, but what of the patient as a human being? In fact, none of the medications being used and none which might have been used for additional complications would have restored Mr. Gage to reasonable health. None would have restored even a minimal personhood, for his capacities for self-awareness and control, interpersonal relations and communication were beyond recovery.

The key concept, "reasonable benefit," must be interpreted in terms of persons and not simply in terms of diseases. For Mr. Gage medications once ordinary had now become heroic. Because of this, the family believed and Dr. Osborn concurred that these treatments were no longer medically or morally mandatory. In fact, their discontinuance had become a moral obligation if faith were to be kept with a husband and father.[6]

Does this mean that anything and everything morally can be omitted in treatment of the terminally ill? Not at all. Our responsibility to care for human life always mandates that we meet certain basic comfort needs: cleanliness, warmth, the easing of bodily positions, and freedom from undue pain or suffering.

Undergirding these ways of caring, there is the responsibility to be with the dying one in love, concern, and physical presence. While the Gage family was convinced of the morality of withdrawing those measures which had become heroic, they were as equally convinced of the importance of these measures of caring which are always obligatory.

Who Decides?

At stake in the situation of John Gage was not only the question "what ought to be done?" but also "who has the right to decide?" Consider those who were involved—or might have been —in the decisions.[7]

First, there was *the patient.* As a general rule, patients themselves ought to have highest priority in deciding those significant actions affecting their lives. But when those decisions about John Gage were called for, he was incapable of communicating. What then? In one way, at least, he was indirectly but crucially involved: his family knew well the values, feelings, and convictions about death and dying he had expressed while still in health. Indeed, their strongest motivation came from "keeping faith with Dad."

Nevertheless, as viewed by those outside the family, this sometimes appears to be "soft data," and it still leaves the burden of decision to those other than the patient. Somewhat "harder data" about the patient's wishes come in some situations from the execution of a Living Will. The "will," which in recent years has been signed by thousands of Americans, has been distributed by various agencies in two major forms—a secular version and a version which incorporates Christian theology. In both cases it is addressed to the individual's family, physician, minister, and attorney, and its message is a brief statement about the person's desires concerning the manner of death. The will thus conveys the individual's wish that, in the event of a terminal illness wherein there is a loss of the patient's own competence for decision-making and in which the quality of life has seriously and irreversibly eroded, his or her dying not be prolonged by artificial means or heroic measures.

Mr. Gage had not executed a Living Will. Had he done so, it still would not have resolved all of the decisional problems. In the first place, these documents are not legally binding even though signed and witnessed while one is still fully competent. Second, by their very nature they cannot anticipate the specific medical circumstances which any individual might encounter during terminal illness. They must be couched in general terms, and to others must be left the task of responsible interpretation in the patient's particular circumstances. Nevertheless, if Mr. Gage had signed such a document it may well have added weight to the family's arguments, for those to whom it is addressed cannot in conscience completely ignore it.

Increasingly it may be possible for patients, while still in good health, to assure themselves of legally-binding representation during their terminal illnesses. A rather innovative law was enacted in New York some years ago, Section 100-A of the 1966 Mental Hygiene Law. Under this statute an individual can designate another person (or several) to be a court-appointed "Committee of the Person" to act on his or her behalf in the event of mental incompetence. The "Committee" is appointed in the manner in which a will is filed or an executor chosen. It has no authority over property matters, but exists solely to make decisions about how the individual is to be treated as a person. Thus, it could fittingly be used to deal with the mode of medical treatment during the final illness. Had this been available in Mr. Gage's state, perhaps the story of his last months would have been different.[8]

In speaking to the question "who ought to decide?" I have begun with the patient. The patient's rights are primary, and it was highly appropriate that the Gage family kept reminding doctors, nurses, and nursing home administrators that they were trying to carry out John Gage's own wishes. To say this does not mean that the patient's rights are absolute. In perspective of the Judeo-Christian vision, no one has absolute rights over his or her own life. We hold our lives in trust, as gifts of the Creator. Even if not an absolute right, however, the patient's right to decide about his or her body has human primacy. It is a weighty right to be defended when that person is seriously ill and at the mercy of the ministrations of others, however well-intended they may be.

After the patient's rights, it is appropriate that the rights of *family* come next. Normally, as was true in the Gage situation, the family has the most intimate relationships and covenantal loyalties established with the patient. They are in the best position to know the wishes of the one who is now unable to decide. Indeed, Christian theology ascribes high status to the family, not simply as a biological unit for procreation but even more as a moral and covenantal relationship for mutual love and fulfillment. Accordingly, Roman Catholic ethics has enunciated "the principle of subsidiarity," whereby the legitimate decisional rights of smaller social units in a society ought not be usurped by larger and more powerful units.

One considerable advantage for giving high priority to family decisions in cases similar to that of John Gage is simply that this precludes compromising the physician's position. Doctors frequently fear the erosion of trust in other patient relationships were they to withdraw supportive treatments from some of the dying. If, however, physicians made it known that such decisions belonged more appropriately to families than to themselves, it is difficult to see how professional confidence would be undermined. It would very likely be enhanced: families would have the assurance that their prerogatives would not be usurped in critical moments.

If no human rights are absolute however important they be, this is also true of the family's decisional rights. The primary concern is what is best for the patient, and on occasion family judgments become distorted by unresolved emotional problems or unworthy motives. When their relationships with the dying patient have been poor over a period of years, they may experience strong guilt feelings during the terminal illness and insist that the doctors do "everything possible." While this might run exactly counter to what is best for the patient, it could assuage the family's regrets: "we'll make it up to him now."

Occasionally families have unworthy motives which preclude their acting in the patient's best interests. Long illnesses produce weariness with emotional and financial burdens. Emotional weariness in itself is not unworthy—it is completely normal for any who really invest themselves in the dying one and indeed can be a mark of the depth of their caring. Unworthy motivation comes only when the good of the patient largely recedes from the family's vision and self-interest becomes dominant.

Protracted terminal illness might also create an impasse in the family. Already involved in the grief process, the spouse and children might find themselves emotionally incapacitated and unable to decide on behalf of the patient. Or, splits in convictions and feelings among members might occur.

These are reminders that both the rights and abilities of families to decide on behalf of the incompetent patient have their limitations. But, in the absence of the patient's own ability to decide and in the absence of strong counterindications concerning the family's ability to consider the patient's welfare, its decisional rights ought to have highest priority. Such rights flow from the covenant of intimacy which is the nature of the family itself.

In the case of John Gage we have seen the futility of the family's efforts to make the major decisions about his treatment during the greater part of his illness. Special appointments were made for discussion with both Bigtown and Plainville doctors. Meetings with staff persons in both nursing homes were held. Letters were written explaining the family's position and urging that the course of treatment be reconsidered.

The turning point began, significantly enough, through the intervention of another physician. After Dr. Osborn's trip to Plainville, Dr. Blecker indicated willingness to begin a partial medication withdrawal. The family's strong desire that their husband and father be allowed to die in his own town, however, was thwarted by the nursing home's refusal to cooperate.

Mrs. Swan's basic reason for refusal, the same reason given

earlier by Dr. Farber, was that the supportive medications were not heroic and hence withdrawal was not morally justifiable. Here, of course, was a significant disagreement with the family on a substantive issue in medical ethics. But also at stake was the companion question: in situations of conflicting judgments about this type of issue whose decision ought to prevail?

An exceptionless general rule arbitrating such impasses in favor of families cannot be erected at this point. For reasons we have seen, there may be limits to the family's moral right to decide on behalf of its incompetent member. The Gages' frustration, however, was that their rights were being abrogated on what appeared to be inappropriate grounds. No strong sense of guilt clouded their motivations; relationships with the husband and father had been warm and deep. Finances were not a major issue. Though the family was experiencing the grief process over the months of seeing John Gage's personhood destroyed, no emotional incapacitation impeded their abilities to think rationally and weigh alternatives carefully. There was no split among family members about what ought to be done; convictions were unanimous and mutually supportive. But in Bigtown and Plainville they were met with the assumption that the medical professionals, by virtue of role and responsibility, must have the final word in such decisions.

Arguments for *the physician's* right to primary voice in these matters ought not be brushed aside lightly. To be sure (see Chapter Two), the religious aura which has surrounded the professional healer during most of our culture's history complicates rational discussion of the issue, and plaques on waiting room walls still conclude: "He who is a sinner towards his Maker will be defiant toward his doctor."

Nevertheless, several arguments have their own persuasiveness. For one, both by law and prevailing practice, the physician has accepted a responsibility for medical treatment of the patient —a responsibility which could be seriously jeopardized if others tell the doctor what course of treatment to pursue. Further, by professional training, it is argued, physicians are best equipped to make such medical decisions. In addition, the doctor might be more objective about the best interests of the patient than either the conscious patient or the family of an unconscious or incompetent one. William A. Nolen, a practicing physician and popular author, expresses this position. While he admits that physicians ought not be dictators, and while he concedes that there are unfortunate communications gaps with patients, his overall philosophy is clear:

> Let's be candid: Doctors run the world of medicine. We decide who will go to the hospital and who will be treated at home; who will receive what medicine; who will have an operation and who will not. We have all the power. There are valid reasons for this concentration of power. Someone has to be "captain"; otherwise, medical care would become fragmented and potentially dangerous. Physicians, since they have the necessary education and training, are the logical leaders. We are the ones best suited to take ultimate responsibility for patients' care.[9]

However, arguments against the physician's primacy in the decisions we are considering are overriding. Daniel Maguire effectively expresses a viewpoint significantly different from Dr. Nolen's:

> [The doctor] is a person skilled in medical technology. His technical advice on the state of a disease and the prospects of its course are indispensable. His counsel on how to achieve death by choice if that is decided upon is also indispensable. . . . But the choice for death is not his. It is a moral choice involving personal, non-medical factors and values over which the doctor has no special competence. . . .[10]

At stake are both the right to decide and the competence to decide, and they are closely interwoven. What of the competence for such decisions? On this matter, physicians as a group can make no special claims. With rare exceptions, their professional training focuses little if any attention upon the non-biological, personal dimensions of the dying process. Nor does medical school seriously engage the student in the examination of the ethics of decision-making in such situations. Add to this the death-as-medical-failure orientation of numerous practitioners. Also consider physicians' tendency to remove themselves from close contact with the dying patient—not only because those patients who have hope deserve more of their time but also because the dying one constitutes a personal threat.

Dr. Maguire correctly assesses the result: when physicians themselves make the fundamental decisions about whether to withhold or withdraw medical supports in terminal cases those decisions take their basic shape from the doctor's own philosophical-religious orientation and not from strictly medical factors themselves.[11] Earl R. Babbie's comment in his study of medical educators' attitudes makes the point:

> A very religious Catholic physician and a very religious Catholic plumber are both likely to oppose infanticide as immoral. The source of their opposition is to be found in their shared religious perspective, however, not in medicine or in plumbing.[12]

It would be both simplistic and unfair merely to blame those physicians who automatically assume finality of decision about terminal care. Some families do thrust awesome matters onto them, and doctors frequently carry excessively heavy moral burdens as a consequence. A shift away from this pattern would, accordingly, accomplish several things. It would relieve practitioners of weighty moral responsibilities they ought not have to shoulder. It would lessen doctors' worries about the effects of particular decisions upon the trust relationships with their other patients. Most importantly, it would restore to patients and families the freedom to make their own life-and-death decisions, freedoms which now are frequently violated even with the best of intentions.

Of the three physicians who figured most prominently into Mr. Gage's care, only Dr. Osborn departed markedly from the prevailing medical cultural practice in these respects. He was clearly aware that there were medical factors in the case for which his professional competence was called and for which he must bear decisional responsibility. He was equally clear that the basic decisions to be made on John Gage's behalf were not strictly medical ones but were fundamentally ethical, philosophical, and theological. He saw his role as an important consultant to the family in their decision. During the period of Dr. Osborn's involvement he kept in close personal touch with the family as well as with the dying patient.

While much of the interaction about decisions in the case of John Gage was among family members and the physicians, others also played significant roles. *Nurses* and nursing home staff persons entered in.[13] Unfortunately, nurses are not often considered as candidates for important roles in such decision-making. Nurses (still mostly women) are victims of our cultural sexism and in a heavily male-dominated medical world are associated with those aspects of medical care which doctors do not highly esteem. Actually, through more intense involvement with both patient and family, the nurse may be in a better position than the doctor to contribute meaningfully to the basic decisions which must be made. Yet, as the nurse participates, professional skills can provide necessary medical data but the ultimate decisions will still be the results of personal orientations, and here the nurse's role, like the doctor's, is not primary. In the nursing homes in both Bigtown and Plainville, staff members played into the decisional discussions—some of them enabling and insightful, others with discomfort and rigidity. In each case, however, it became clear to the Gage family that the nurses were sharing basic beliefs and value orientations more than technical knowledge. Given the decisions which had to be made, it could not be otherwise.

Clergy, both parish pastors and hospital chaplains, were also involved in the John Gage case. For several reasons, ministers may be in positions to make significant contributions to the decisions about terminal care. Their opportunity for personal involvement with both patient and family is often greater than that of medical professionals. They have been trained to assist persons in making moral decisions; unlike the medical school, the seminary does emphasize ethical reflection and the importance of dealing with the questions of meaning which surround the dying process. Further, the covenant relationship assumed to exist among patient, families, and clergy tends to be more inclusive than that assumed in strictly medical relationships. While inclinations toward spiritualism to the neglect of the body have long plagued religious professionals, concern for the wholeness of human life increasingly characterizes parish ministers as well as chaplains. Indeed, there is evidence that clergy, in comparison with doctors, show significantly more concern about the patient's entire social context.

Yet, there are frequent limitations to clerical effectiveness. Two are particularly prevalent. As we have seen earlier (Chapter Three), both parish ministers and hospital chaplains have tended to accent the priestly sides of their ministries to the neglect of the prophetic dimensions. Though their professional training has made them knowledgeable about ethical reflection, the pressures of surrounding culture and the reward systems of their institutions tend to depreciate their use of these insights. Hence, many clergy are unaccustomed to affirming, much less asserting, their own potentially important contributions to such moral decision-making. Related to this is a second reason. In practice, physicians frequently treat chaplains and pastors as having rather incidental roles to play in these moral decisions, if not in the entire healing process. And, having accepted somewhat uncritically the cultural evaluations of the two professions, some clergy acquiesce too quickly to the doctor's judgment. Witness this not infrequent occurrence: the minister is making a patient call in the hospital and the two are in the midst of significant conversation; the physician enters; the minister readily (and expectedly) defers, leaves the room so that "more important" things can happen, and returns at "a more convenient time."

In spite of these limiting temptations, clergy often do make notable contributions to the moral decisions which surround the dying. They tend to be more qualified by both training and orientation to see the patient's situation in its broadest relational context. Numerous hospital chaplains have forged effective collegial relationships with the medical staff and are respected for their abilities to play crucial roles in such decisional processes. The same is true of many parish pastors, particularly when working with medical staff with whom they are well-acquainted. Just as other professionals involved in basic terminal care decisions, however, the clergy have an important auxiliary role but not the primary decisional right.

None of the ministers involved with the Gages assumed such a right; each took a supportive and enabling role. The two parish clergy in Plainville expressed primarily priestly functions, seeking to sustain the family members but avoiding ethical counseling and advocacy. The chaplains in Metropolis, no less priestly, also willingly explored the decisional issue with the family and helped to facilitate its course in the hospital there.

Another possibility in the roster of those involved in decisions about the terminally ill remains: *a committee*. Some hospitals have established them for this purpose. Hennepin County Medical Center in Minneapolis is one. Its "Thanatology Committee" includes physicians, chaplains, nurses, and hospital social workers. This group considers specific terminal cases in which difficult decisions must be faced. Recommendations about possible courses of action are then made to appropriate staff members and to family members, who may be included in the discussions. Hospital policies dealing with care of the dying are also grist for the committee's mill.

Two distinct benefits accrue from the functioning of such a committee, particularly when there are no near relatives of the dying patient (a not altogether unusual situation in a general hospital). For one thing, decisions of such fundamental importance ought to be made communally and not unilaterally, and the committee's work expresses this principle. Also, such communal decisions ought to represent varying vantage points expressed by persons who stand in different role relations to the patient.

Even the best of committees always bring problems, however, and this type is no exception. Committees set up to deal with questions surrounding the dying ought always to guard against the temptation to usurp the decisional rights of the conscious patient or of the family of a comatose or incompetent one. They ought to function in advisory capacities in all but the exceptional case wherein hospital staff persons must act on behalf of the patient. Care must be exercised in committee composition and dynamics. It is more convenient, perhaps, to have only hospital staff represented, but the need for family and "public" input is crucial. Further, given the medical ethos which still obtains, there is the danger of automatic physician dominance in the committee's work. Private hospitals with particular religious orientations toward death questions must take care not to impose those views upon non-consenting patients. Finally, the temptation toward bureaucratization and abstraction of deeply personal decisions must be resisted.

The risks are present. Yet the fruits already borne by some death-and-dying committees warrants a very hopeful judgment about their future possibilities.

What About the Law?

American law regarding direct or active euthanasia is clear: it is first-degree murder. Unfortunately, the law itself takes no account of a merciful motive. However, prosecutors have been reluctant to indict and juries reluctant to convict. In the few convictions of murder and the somewhat larger number of homicide convictions in direct euthanasia cases, those who administer the law have been notably lenient in meting out punishment. The theory of the law and the application of the law have been quite different.

However, our concern in this chapter is not with direct but

with indirect or passive euthanasia. And, because the word *euthanasia* in any context may frighten and mislead, let us again rephrase the matter: where does the law currently stand regarding cooperating with the dying process rather than medically resisting it in terminal cases? regarding the omission of heroic treatments for the dying?

Prior to the lower court's decision in the case of Karen Ann Quinlan late in 1975, several factors seemed to indicate that the legality of passive euthanasia increasingly was being recognized.[14] No American court had successfully ordered a legally competent adult without dependent children to undergo medical treatment, even when the refusal of such treatment certainly meant an earlier death. Further, the patient's rights movement was gaining force. Numerous hospitals had adopted the "Patient's Bill of Rights" recommended by the American Hospital Association, a statement which contained this provision: "The patient has the right to refuse treatment to the extent permitted by law, and to be informed of the medical consequences of his action." To be sure, "the extent permitted by law" remained somewhat unclear, since no state had yet spelled this out by statute. Yet, case law, the law as applied in the courts, virtually always hinged upon "prevailing standards of medical practice," and those standards had increasingly recognized the morality of refusal—by and on behalf of the terminally ill. In addition, it was being argued that since American legal principle guarantees personal autonomy as long as the individual does not jeopardize the rights of others, this principle protects one's right to refuse consent to medical treatment. An appropriate corollary to this appeared to be the family's right to decide, with medical advice, on behalf of a permanently incompetent patient.

Then came November 10, 1975, and the decision of Judge Robert Muir, Jr. in the Morris County Superior Court of New Jersey, a decision which brought confusion to both the moral and legal scenes. It was a classic case. Never before had passive euthanasia so clearly been tested in the courts. It was a tragic case. Karen Quinlan had suffered massive brain damage the previous April and had been in "a persistent vegetative state" ever since with a contorted and emaciated body and with no physicians holding out reasonable hope for meaningful recovery. The financial costs, moreover, were astronomical and were being borne by society. And the moral clarity of the case was convincing to many. Karen's devoted and devout Catholic parents were backed by the moral support of their priest, their bishop, and papal teaching. Thwarted in their attempts to have her respirator withdrawn, they were now appealing to the court for legal permission to do so.

Given the courts' strong reluctance to weaken the principle of the protection of innocent life, the decision may not have been surprising. Yet, it was disheartening. It failed to distinguish between "killing" and "allowing to die," and in so doing firmly equated legal homicide and passive euthanasia. It declared that the distinction between extraordinary and ordinary medical measures was not a viable legal distinction.

Furthermore, Judge Muir ruled that the decision concerning when to stop medical treatments was a medical decision to be made by medical professionals. This was doubly unfortunate. For one thing it involved a basic confusion between facts and values (Chapter One). It confused the question of Karen's medical prognosis (a matter of scientific estimate for which the physicians, indeed, alone were competent) with the question of what ought to be done in light of that prognosis (a value question concerning which physicians have no special competence or right to determine). In addition, the claim that this was "a medical decision" undercut the family's basic decisional rights—with potentially serious consequences for the rights of future patients and families in every sort of decision about their medical treatment.

Finally, the first Quinlan decision rested upon a biological absolutism: an absolute commitment to the sanctity of biological human life regardless of its personal quality. Said the judge, "The single most important temporal quality Karen Ann Quinlan has is life," a statement difficult to understand considering this woman's persistent vegetative state for the seven previous months. In any event, that a biological absolutism was basic to this legal decision seems indicated by a hypothetical role reversal: had it been the *doctors* who had wanted to *remove* the respirator, and had it been *Mr. and Mrs. Quinlan* who had wanted the respirator to *remain,* would the judge still have ruled that this was a medical decision to be made by the medical professionals? I believe not.[15]

Then came March 31, 1976 and the ruling of the Supreme Court of New Jersey on the Quinlan case. It is no exaggeration to view this as a landmark ruling. Chief Justice Richard Hughes spoke for a unanimous court in reversing virtually every major point of the lower court's decision.

- The constitutional right to privacy in such medical decisions was recognized: "We think that the State's interest *contra* weakens and the individual's right to privacy grows as the degree of bodily invasion increases and the prognosis dims. Ultimately there comes a point at which the individual's rights overcome the State interest." [16]

- The decision concerning whether or not to remove the artificial life supports was not simply "a medical decision": "Determinations as to these must, in the ultimate, be responsive not only to the concepts of medicine but also to the common moral judgment of the community at large." [17]

- Such a decision to refuse to prolong the process of dying was not a threat to the religious and moral commitment to life: "We think these attitudes represent a balanced implementation of a profoundly realistic perspective on the meaning of life and death and that they respect the whole Judeo-Christian tradition of regard for human life." [18]

- The distinction between ordinary and extraordinary medical measures was a viable distinction, and the distinction depended more basically upon the situation of the patient than upon the technology itself: " . . . the use of the same respirator or like support could be considered 'ordinary' in the context of the possibly curable patient but 'extraordinary' in the context of the forced sustaining by cardio-respiratory processes of an irreversibly doomed patient." [19]

• Passive euthanasia was not to be confused, either legally or morally, with homicide: ". . . the ensuing death would not be homicide but rather expiration from existing natural causes. . . . There is a real and in this case determinative distinction between the unlawful taking of the life of another and the ending of artificial life-support systems as a matter of self-determination." [20]

• In prescribing a hospital "Ethics Committee," the court recognized that decisions of this sort should be made with communal consultation. In addition, however, by returning the guardianship of Karen Quinlan's person to her father, the court recognized that the family had the final decisional right, given medical agreement "that there is no reasonable possibility of Karen's ever emerging from her present comatose condition. . . ." [21]

• Finally and fundamentally the court recognized that this type of moral decision was appropriately made with regard to the quality of meaningful personal life rather than upon an unyielding commitment to biological existence as such: "The evidence in this case convinces us that the focal point of decision should be the prognosis as to the reasonable possibility of return to cognitive and sapient life, as distinguished from the forced continuance of that biological vegetative existence to which Karen seems to be doomed." [22]

The Karen Quinlan case as decided by the Supreme Court of New Jersey provides both welcome and highly significant clarification for the major legal issues surrounding passive euthanasia, allowing the dying to die. Its effect on moral attitudes and professional practices in our society will take years to assess, perhaps. Nevertheless, had the ruling come some months earlier, the case of John Gage might have looked different.

The Right to Decide

In the annals of ethics a "right" is a power reserved to the person such that he or she can justly demand that it not be interfered with or taken away. When we speak of rights we ought also to speak of the other side of the coin: duties. The two are correlative. One person's rights involve acknowledgment of the claims of others.

A Christian faith based upon a radical monotheism has difficulty talking about any absolute human rights. Absolutes belong to God alone. Thus, even the conscious dying patient does not have an absolute right to decide about his or her body, nor does the family have that kind of right over the dwindling life of the incompetent patient. Our rights over our bodies exist in relation to our duties or responsibilities to the Creator who has given us life. But that Creator is also our Redeemer who, through the gift of faith, might yet save us from anxious biological idolatries which insist upon the continuation of physiological life signs at any price, regardless of that life's quality.

When momentous decisions during sad terminal illnesses must be made on behalf of the patient incapable of deciding, a good general principle is this: they ought to be made communally by those bound in special covenants of responsibility to the patient. The corollary is this: the weight of power in the decisional process ought to depend upon the nature of the particular covenantal relationship.

Normally, the covenants of marriage and family bear the greatest intimacy and responsibility. Members of these covenants have rights of decision which ought not be interfered with nor taken away. There are, to be sure, exceptions—when the covenant of responsibility has been torn by estrangement or when it is clear beyond reasonable doubt that the family's decision runs counter to the known values and wishes of the patient. But in the more usual situation, as was true with the Gages, such exceptions are not present. Then the family's decision ought still to be made communally, drawing upon the counsel of physician and nurse, chaplain and pastor, perhaps hospital social worker, and often close friends. These persons, too, are bound to the patient in varying covenants of responsibility and rightfully deserve to contribute to the decision even if it is not, in the final analysis, theirs to make.

Epilog

John Gage was not allowed to die in his home town, nor in the larger community nearby in his home state. To keep faith with him his family moved him several hundred miles away. Their natural grief processes over the progressive personal death of a beloved member were compounded by deep frustration over the obstacles to his dignified release. They had to undertake the additional weight of planning and strategizing, arguing and persuading. It need not have been so, but our society is still in its adolescence in coping with the meanings and processes of death.

The issues in this case retain their measure of human ambiguity, and my ethical comments show their obvious bias. But I have seriously attempted to be fair in describing the positions held and actions taken by the various people, all well-intentioned, whose names have been fictitiously represented in the foregoing account. "John Gage" was my father-in-law, and "Jane" and I were having our turn at Dad's bedside when his physiological death mercifully came in the middle of that August night. Her words of relief were utterly appropriate in that sorrowful-yet-triumphant moment: "Daddy, we finally won."

Persons, Values, and Medicine in the Century's Fourth Quarter

Symptoms of Malaise

While the beginning of the century's fourth quarter is an exciting time in medicine, it is not a particularly comfortable one. As in so many other fields the excitement is technological, but the malaise is personal and interpersonal. There is an ironic symbolism in the juxtaposition: the totally-implantable artificial heart is virtually upon us, yet more medical professionals and laity are disappointed with health care than at any other time within memory. Consider some of the symptoms:

Symptom: the malpractice insurance crisis. The quarter's opening year saw doctor slowdowns and strikes in locations from Alaska to Florida and New York to California. Malpractice insurance rates rose geometrically and, in some cases, became prohibitive. Lawsuits, once a rarity, were the order of the day. A national study discovered one out of every seven general surgeons facing a malpractice complaint in 1975. A California survey indicated that never had there been a million-dollar judgment until 1967, but there were thirteen such judgments in the years 1973 to 1975 alone.[1]

Symptom: mistrust of medical research. In the quarter's opening year the editor of the prestigious *New England Journal of Medicine* said, "In the name of ethics, anti-intellectualism and anti-science are encouraged, hostility to medicine is nourished, clinical investigation is compromised if not castrated and the cause of probity itself is harmed." ² Dr. Franz J. Ingelfinger was criticizing those "activist groups" who he believed were exploiting the recent concern for medical ethics and frightening the public to a point where experimental medicine was hamstrung by unwilling participants and a bureaucracy of consent committees.

Symptom: lack of communication between ethicists and physicians. Toward the beginning of the century's fourth quarter, Dr. Irvine H. Page, editor of *Modern Medicine,* wrote in frustration, "What do such terms as myth, distributive justice, situational ethics, structural-functionalism, manifest function, societal guidance, and identity mean to you?" Doctors, he maintained, have had little training in ethics but now are expected to grasp the ethical subtleties of all the medical issues with which they are dealing. "Most physicians do not understand whether ethical decisions are made on the basis of a majority vote, absolute authority of the Church or State, the power of bias, the concept of survival, or simple pragmatism. . . . Perhaps you will understand a little better why many of us are groping and baffled." ³

Symptom: increasing impersonality of physician-patient relationships. After describing three cases in which a breakdown in doctor-patient communication caused serious distress for the patients, Dr. William A. Nolen summarized: "All three of these patients received proper, scientific medical care from their doctors, and yet every one of them was mistreated. They, and their families, needed and deserved more—and more prompt—information than they got. These patients were all victims of what might be called 'the doctor-patient communication gap.' This gap, in my opinion, is one of the most serious problems in medicine." ⁴

Symptom: serious problems in the cost, quality, and distribution of medical care. The cost problems were becoming enormous. In the two decades between 1950 and 1970 there was a four hundred percent increase in medical expenditures. By the beginning of the fourth quarter Americans were spending fifty-six percent more on medical services than they had only five years earlier, and approximately half of the people who filed pleas of personal bankruptcy did so because of medical debts. The cost increases had far surpassed the inflation rate. Catastrophic illnesses continued to destroy family financial patterns, so that Oscar Wilde's statement had new pertinence: not only are we living beyond our means but we are also dying beyond our means.

The quality of medical care is a legitimate concern. Undoubtedly the American medical system still leads the world in the quality of medical research and therapeutic crisis care. Yet the statistics which trace infant mortality, life expectancy, and other indices of overall health care in the United States are sobering when compared with those of other industrialized nations. We do not rank well. In spite of the enormous advances in medical biology and the marked decrease of infectious diseases, a whole host of "diseases of civilization" (ulcers, heart disease, high blood pressure) are increasing. Our medical system, for all of its virtues, simply has not placed a premium on preventive medicine.

Marks of the distribution and accessibility problems are becoming well-known. There are four times as many physicians in some geographic areas as there are in others. Small communities in many parts of the country are without doctors. Physicians have specialized in numbers disproportionate to the health needs of the public. For example, an excessive supply of surgeons seems to beget an excessive number of surgical procedures—not out of the distorted motivations of knife-happy and greedy surgeons, but simply because one tends to do what one has been especially trained to do. But paramount among the distribution problems is the cruel lack of medical services for the poor and for many members of ethnic and racial minorities. We have long known in the abstract that the poor are much more likely to be chronically ill and the chronically ill to be poor, but we have done little to change that picture.

Some Reflections about Persons, Love, and Justice

To the foregoing symptoms of malaise is our current health care patterns, numerous responses are warranted. Many of these should be policy recommendations and programmatic outlines. Take but one example, the malpractice insurance problem. Thoughtful response to this demands consideration of a whole range of alternatives: state-supported insurance funds with limited insurance fees; legal ceilings on malpractice awards; limitations of contingency fees for attorneys; redefinitions of malpractice to cover incompetence and negligence but not medical misfortune; statutes of limitation for the pressing of malpractice suits; arbitration panels; more effective professional self-policing; and basic changes in health care delivery system. Each of these possibilities should be weighed.

But such is not our task here. Ours is at once more limited and more basic. It is simply to argue that while the solutions to our medical care problems do indeed demand policy changes, new programs, and altered structures, they *also* require changes in attitudes, in values, in ways of looking at ourselves and at the world. In short, our problems in medical care are just as theological as they are economic, political, and technological.

While numerous theological themes would be appropriate, consider just three—personhood, love, and justice. Each interweaves with the others, and together they illustrate the relevance of theological reflection to the problems at hand.

First, our beliefs about the human person. Biblical thought knows little if anything about the solitary individual. The scriptural roots of Judeo-Christian thought typically see the person as a self-in-community. We know what it means to be a self only in relationship with others. We are quite literally humanized through communication and dialog. We live in communities, and communities live in us. Most fundamentally we are called into personhood through communion with God. In the Garden of Eden narrative the Genesis writer puts its quite simply: God speaks of the lower animals as "they," but addresses Adam and Eve as "you."

Consider our notions of love and justice. Again, our biblical heritage knows little if anything about the private and sentimental notions of love which are bawled at us over millions of loudspeakers daily. Nor does that heritage endorse a notion of justice which is the social arrangement conceived and maintained by those who have the power to do so. These common distortions of love and justice have one basic flaw: the two are split apart. The result, as Reinhold Niebuhr characteristically put it, is this: love without justice becomes mere sentimentality, and justice without love becomes only another balance of power.[5]

But when the two concepts are held together in mutual and creative tension, another picture emerges. Love, in Christian perspective, is that self-giving and self-fulfilling relationship which binds creatures together in acceptance and harmony, and the created with the Creator. The paradigm of love is Jesus Christ. But this kind of love always demands justice, for love works toward fulfillment of persons, and persons are very social beings. Justice is that social arrangement which, given the limitations imposed by both human finitude and human sin, best offers that fulfillment for all persons. And the norm of love never allows us to be satisfied with any particular expression of justice. Our social organizations and structures could always be more fair, more fulfilling, more accessible to all than they presently are. Love constantly reminds us of that.

This brief theological excursion, abstract though it may seem initially, raises issues of utmost practicality about health care and the symptoms of malaise which presently plague us. Consider again the malpractice insurance problem.

This syndrome may be alleviated by some of the policy and program measures listed earlier, but its basic causes do not lie in the absence of award limitations and arbitration panels. More basically the causes lie in the self-perceptions of health professionals and patients and in what has been happening to the relationships between these groups. The root issues are personhood, love, and justice.

Commenting on the problems underlying soaring malpractice rates, Dr. Judah Folkman of Harvard Medical School perceives something of this. Doctors, he said, must think of their patients as persons and not simply as medical consumers. They must remember that good medicine begins and ends with compassion. Indeed, studies do show that patients who have been treated with compassion are unlikely to sue, whatever the medical results of their treatment, while patients who feel themselves slighted tend to express their dissatisfaction through the courts.[6]

Dr. Folkman is counseling more than an enlightened self-interest. He does not mean that doctors ought to be compassionate *in order to* avoid malpractice suits. They ought to be compassionate because good medical care depends upon it, and malpractice suits are minimal in good medical care.

Nevertheless, the issue of compassion in the professional-patient relationship needs a second look. At first thought it would seem that compassion is simply an expression of love. The compassionate doctor is one who treats the patient as a person, not simply as a case or as a medical consumer. And persons have hopes and joys, fears and anxieties about their health. The physician needs to participate in those dimensions of a patient's life, at least to the extent that they bear upon good medical care. And the patient needs and deserves honest and open communication. Such seem to be marks of love expressed as compassion.

But another term is needed in this equation: justice. If love without justice becomes sentimentality, surely compassion without justice becomes paternalism, however well-intended it may be. Medical care in our society—even at its most compassionate— has long shown strong signs of paternalism. It has been the physician's assumed right not only to prescribe the cure but also to define what health is, what diseases are, and which diseases call for treatment.

Granted, the rise in malpractice claims is due in part to the higher, sometimes unrealistic, expectations of the public about medicine. Thanks to the mass media, the public is more medically-informed than ever, and thanks to Marcus Welby at times it has almost perfectionistic expectations of medical treatment. Further, the rise in claims is due in part to underemployed lawyers who sense a lucrative field here, particularly as no-fault auto insurance diminishes another area of their practice. But beyond these, malpractice claims appear to uncover an underlying frustration: patient powerlessness.

Justice, however, calls for the abandonment of paternalistic models and for the appropriation of more participatory models of medicine. Indeed, one of the marks of justice is equal access— the possibility of equal access by all persons to those decisions which vitally affect them and to those resources which are necessary for human fulfillment. A more participatory medicine will involve changes both in self-images and in perceptions of the task. It will call for physicians who willingly relinquish high-priestly identities and embrace the creative tension between the prophetic and the priestly (Chapter Two). However, participatory medicine will also involve changes in our perception of the task of health care.

Pause for a moment to retrace the steps of this illustration. The main point is that the pressing problems in current medical care are theological in nature as well as economic, political, and technological. Malpractice problems are a case in point. New insurance and claims structures alone will help, but by themselves they will not get at the underlying ailment. At a deeper level is the need for compassion in medical relationships. But compassion as an expression of love must be mated with justice, and justice presses us toward a vision of more participatory medicine. This, in turn, means among other things that patients and public as well as health professionals participate in the definitions of what health and disease really are.

Doctors and medical laity alike typically evaluate the quality of health care in terms of the success of the treatment given to part of an individual's anatomy. Physicians John G. Bruhn and Douglas C. Smith recognize the inadequacy of this: "Many health professionals are reluctant to accept the medical importance of social and psychological aspects of the patient's life. Apparently, they either do not know or are indifferent to how often the recovery of health depends on the presence or absence of social support, hope, or life satisfaction."[7]

Precisely this broadened redefinition of health was the aim of the World Health Organization, as we noted in Chapter One. "Health," said WHO, "is a state of complete physical, mental, and social well-being and not merely the absence of disease or infirmity." The definition quite appropriately points to the wholeness of the person and recognizes that this wholeness is not only a unity of body and spirit but also the harmony of person and community.

But here we run into trouble. By such an expanded definition we seem to include everything related to human happiness under the rubric of health. The consequence of this would seem to be the assignment of the medical professional as the gate-keeper for our total well-being, a role which would further alienate the patient who felt his or her own lack of power in the relationship. Perceptive critics of the WHO definition have recognized this. Daniel Callahan summarizes his major objections: since health is only part of life and the achievement of health only part of human happiness, medicine's role ought to be recognized as a legitimately limited one; further, by putting all human virtues and vices into the categories of health and illness, we undercut human freedom, responsibility, and morality.[8] Robert M. Veatch notes, not without seriousness, that such an encompassing definition of health "means that, in effect, the medical professional is the one to turn to for technically competent help in such failures in well-being as marriage problems, poverty, and unanswered prayers."[9]

It looks like a dilemma. If we wish to keep the authority and tasks of the medical professionals within appropriate boundaries, we end up with a definition of health which is excessively individualistic and physiological. Contrarily, if we embrace a more inclusive definition of health, we have made an impossibly broad definition and given the medical professionals license to be the arbiters of life itself.

The objections are valid warnings, but they do not necessarily impale us on the horns of a dilemma. For several reasons a broad definition of health is quite compatible with an appropriately limited role for medical professionals. First, medicine does not constitute the whole of health. Health *is* a positive state of well-being, and there is theological precedent for seeing it in this way. The linguistic roots for *health, wholeness,* and *salvation* are common roots. There is no necessary reason why the medical professions should claim—or be saddled with—authority for the whole of human health. Secretaries and electricians, plumbers and kindergarten teachers, housewives and househusbands have important responsibilities in the enterprise of human wholeness.

Further, the claim that a broad definition of health undercuts moral responsibility needs a second look. True, in recent decades our society has moved more and more types of human behavior and condition out of the categories of irresponsibility or sin and into the category of illness. And we tend not to blame one who is ill. But a blanket notion of "no-fault illness" is itself questionable. The more we learn about the sociology of medicine, the more we learn that the nature of sick roles is as much sociologically determined as physiologically determined. Our society typically removes the one labeled as sick not only from normal day-to-day responsibilities; we also remove from that person the responsibility for the illness in the first place. It is questionable, in light of our increasing knowledge of the psychosomatic dimensions of illness, whether responsibility for *all* kinds of physical sickness ought to be removed from personal accountability. Granted that relatives, friends, and the wider society must share responsibility because of their rejecting attitudes, nevertheless it *may* well be that Uncle Archibald is as responsible for his attention-getting physical ailment as he would be for an attention-getting bank robbery.

There is one more reason for staying with the broader definition of health. The appropriate constraints upon the authority of medical professionals will come not only from definitions of health, important though they may be. At least as significant will be the daily interaction of people in medical situations. Patients and families and members of the public at large who take more active responsibilities will provide countervailing power in the clinic and hospital, relieving medical professionals of burdens they should neither be required nor allowed to bear alone.

Consider once again our understanding of personhood. Earlier we noted (Chapter One) that in contrast with biblical perceptions of person as self-in-community, our society has been deeply affected by philosophical and political individualism. According to this view, the individual is the basic unit of reality. Relationships with others, communities, society as a whole— these are accidental and not essential to the individual. While, in its extreme forms, such individualism is both theological and socio-psychological nonsense, parts of this philosophy have brought significant benefits to this society—particularly our concerns for individual freedom and autonomy and our remarkable impetus to technological development.

But in our health care arrangements we are now reaping a rather stunted harvest from the individualistic notion of the person.[10] Health care arrangements take their essential form in a one-to-one contract between two individuals, and the role of the wider community is incidental at best or suspect at worst. (Thus we pay our private practitioners substantially more than our public health physicians, and thus we find brain surgery a more appropriate form of medicine than the prevention of lead poisoning.) Individualism in medicine can mean that medical service is offered in a narrowly technical and fragmented manner. (One of the major impediments to good health care for many is their lack of knowledge of what medical treatment they need or how to find it.) Individualism makes of the sick community a series of individual patients unrelated to each other. (This undercuts the transmission of shared experience among patients and also thwarts the organization of consumer pressure.) And, of course, the individualistic medical model keeps many people from adequate medicine. (Either they lack the money to make the contract, or the entrepreneurial model of physician distribution has left their community with inadequate services.)

The medical situation in China is instructive, by way of contrast. There the burden of proof is shifted. In our society the main responsibility is the doctor's—to cure the patient. In China, the main responsibility lies with each person—to stay well, to protect the health of the neighbor, and to participate in the social organization of health care activity.[11]

Granted, the social and intellectual history of China is far different from ours. There, while individuality has been encouraged in certain respects, individualism has been utterly foreign. The person in China is first and foremost the member of the group, and it is the individual's main responsibility to work for the common good, never for his or her own private interests. In their analysis of the Chinese health care system, Victor and Ruth Sidel recognize that to Western eyes there appears to be considerable coercion in this approach. But, they say, "in the Chinese context, it appears quite different. Where society rather than the individual is viewed as the basic unit . . . the actions of any individual are always seen as irrevocably tied to the well-being of the larger group."[12]

China's brand of socialism would be unacceptable to most of us. Indeed, viewing the group as *the* basic social unit has as many inherent problems as viewing the individual as the basic unit. But if there is falsity in both approaches, there is also truth in each. We are persons-in-community — neither individuals for whom community is a dispensable luxury, nor individuals whose meaning and purpose is found only in the larger society. Underneath the malpractice insurance malaise lies a skewed notion of personhood in our society. Even while it carries some important truth, its heavy tilt in the direction of individualism has nurtured a no-fault notion of illness in the minds of many patients, has placed unfair and unrealistic expectations upon medical professionals, and has precluded the strong development of health maintenance and preventive care. Our doctrine of personhood has as much practical importance to the malpractice issue as does legislative action. The two are intertwined and both need serious attention. But the former is fundamental.

We could have chosen examples other than malpractice insurance to illustrate the point. Indeed, other examples might have been even more significant. What, for instance, of the goals needed in a national health care policy—universality, accessibility, comprehensiveness of care, accountability to the public, equitable financing, continual planning? [13] What of the relation of health care in America to the drastic health care needs of the Third World? [14] But the main point is the same: in each instance of significant medical issues we are driven back to our philosophical, indeed, theological notions about such matters as love, justice, and personhood. And as we begin to examine these basic assumptions we begin to see more clearly how all of the problems are, at the bottom, tied together. The issues beneath the surface of the malpractice insurance problem are the same root issues underlying national health policy and the relation of American medicine to medicine in Bangladesh in an interdependent world.

If, in the century's third quarter our preoccupation was with medical technology, its amazing possibilities and incumbent problems, these issues will not disappear in the fourth quarter. But in the fourth quarter, our focus of attention surely needs expansion to include these fundamental theological issues which, for good or for ill, give shape to the manner in which we pursue our common medical enterprise.

Exodus, Liberation, and Health

Our theological heritage is rich with insights which might yet reorient our ways of perceiving our current health care situation. Professor Walter Brueggemann appropriately reminds us that the primal event of the Old Testament—the exodus—has a direct relevance.[15] Reading the story as a case study in health care, one can assume that Pharaoh undoubtedly controlled all the resources of technical medicine of that time and place, but he shared them with none of the Israelite slaves. Medicine was only for those who belonged. The Israelites, presumably, had no right to it—it was a privilege which was not theirs.

But then the liberating God becomes real in the experience of the Israelites, and their liberation from bondage becomes a primal event of healing. So throughout the Old Testament liberation, empowerment, restoration, and reconciliation are all dimensions of healing. And the history of Israel displays that perennial tension between kings and prophets. The former retain for themselves the resources for health and well-being and dispense them according to their own self-interest. The latter insist that God's healing cannot be controlled in this exclusive manner.

So it is in the New Testament. The chief priests and scribes had carefully delimited the blessings of well-being and presumed to assign them to those with the right qualifications. Jesus, however, inaugurated a new health care system. It infuriated the elite. It seemed to violate all reasonable and respectable standards. But the blind did receive their sight, and the lame did walk, and lepers were cleansed . . . and the poor did find good news.

Health care does involve programs and procedures, but it is always more. It involves the fundamental ways in which we perceive our world—and the One who gives ultimate meaning to our world.

Notes

CHAPTER 1: Underlying Issues

1. Charles M. Schulz, *Who Do You Think You Are, Charlie Brown?* (New York: Fawcett World Library, 1958, 1959, 1960, 1961). By permission of Charles M. Schulz.

2. See for example Joseph Fletcher, *Morals and Medicine* (Boston: Beacon Press, 1960); Paul Ramsey, *The Patient as Person* (New Haven: Yale University Press, 1970); Harmon L. Smith, *Ethics and the New Medicine* (Nashville: Abingdon Press, 1970); Kenneth Vaux, *Biomedical Ethics* (New York: Harper & Row, 1974); and my own *Human Medicine* (Minneapolis: Augsburg Publishing House, 1973).

3. See James M. Gustafson, *Can Ethics Be Christian?* (Chicago: University of Chicago Press, 1975), esp. Chaps. 1 and 2; see also my book *Moral Nexus: Ethics of Christian Identity and Community* (Philadelphia: The Westminster Press, 1971).

4. See Chauncey D. Leake, "The Humanistic Tradition in the Health Professions," in Maurice B. Visscher (ed.), *Humanistic Perspectives in Medical Ethics* (Buffalo: Prometheus Books, 1972), pp. 20f.

5. "A Definition of Irreversible Coma," in Donald R. Cutler (ed.), *Updating Life and Death* (Boston: Beacon Press, 1968, 1969), p. 55.

6. Robert M. Veatch points this out clearly in reference to the Harvard Ad Hoc Committee. See his "Generalization of Expertise," *Hastings Center Studies,* Vol. 1, No. 2 (1973), p. 30.

7. See also my *Human Medicine,* Chap. One, for additional discussions of this issue and of health and wholeness.

8. See Seward Hiltner, "The Bible Speaks to the Health of Man," in Dale White (ed.), *Dialogue in Medicine and Theology* (Nashville: Abingdon Press, 1967, 1968).

9. Although he is critical of the WHO definition, Daniel Callahan rightly recognizes its virtues as well in "The WHO Definition of 'Health,' " *Hastings Center Studies,* Vol. 1, No. 3 (1973), p. 77.

10. Mervyn Susser, "Ethical Components in the Definition of Health," *International Journal of Health Services,* Vol. 4, No. 3 (1974), p. 541.

11. See Paul Ramsey, *The Patient as Person,* Chap. 1.

12. See Joseph Fletcher, "New Beginnings in Life: A Theologian's Response," in Michael P. Hamilton (ed.), *The New Genetics and the Future of Man* (Grand Rapids: William B. Eerdmans, 1972), pp. 81ff.

13. See Peter Steinfels, "Individualism—No Exit," and Peter Sidgwick, "Medical Individualism," in *Hastings Center Studies,* Vol. 2, No. 3 (1974). Cf. Steven Lukes, *Individualism* (New York: Harper and Row, 1973), esp. pp. 45ff.

14. Process theologians, particularly, have articulated this type of position. See, for example, Norman Pittenger, *The Christian Church as Social Process* (Philadelphia: The Westminster Press, 1971).

15. From *Our Town* by Thornton Wilder. Copyright 1938, 1957 by Thornton Wilder. By permission of Harper & Row.

CHAPTER 2: Personhood of the Physician

1. See my *Human Medicine* (Minneapolis: Augsburg Publishing House, 1973), Chap. Eight, for a fuller development of this theme.

2. For numerous insights concerning the secularization of medicine, I am indebted to Roy Branson, "The Secularization of American Medicine," *Hastings Center Studies,* Vol. 1, No. 2 (1973), pp. 17ff.

3. See Edmund D. Pellegrino, "Educating the Humanist Physician: An Ancient Ideal Reconsidered," *Journal of the American Medical Association,* Vol. 227, No. 11 (March 18, 1974), p. 1291.

4. Edmund D. Pellegrino, in an address to the American Society of Christian Ethics, Knoxville, Tennessee, January 17, 1975.

5. Quoted in John G. Bruhn and Douglas C. Smith, "Social Ethics for Medical Educators," in Maurice Visscher (ed.), *Humanistic Perspectives in Medical Ethics* (Buffalo: Prometheus Books, 1972), p. 289.

6. See Robert M. Veatch, "Models for Ethical Medicine in a Revolutionary Age," *Hastings Center Report,* Vol. 2, No. 3 (June 1972).

7. Renee C. Fox, "Is There a 'New' Medical Student? A Comparative View of Medical Socialization in the 1950s and the 1970s," in Laurence R. Tancredi (ed.), *Ethics of Health Care* (Washington: National Academy of Sciences, 1974), p. 199.

8. *Ibid.,* p. 211.

9. *Ibid.,* p. 214.

10. Chauncey D. Leake, "The Humanistic Tradition in the Health Professions," in Visscher, *op. cit.,* pp. 2ff.

11. See Albert R. Jonsen and Andre E. Hellegers, "Conceptual Foundations for an Ethics of Medical Care," in Tancredi, *op. cit.,* p. 7.

CHAPTER 3: Personhood of the Chaplain

1. Thomas F. Pettigrew, *Christians in Racial Crisis* (Public Affairs Press, 1959).

2. Lawrence E. Holst and Harold P. Kurtz (eds.), *Toward a Creative Chaplaincy* (Charles C. Thomas: Springfield, Ill., 1973), p. 3.

3. Fred W. Reid, Jr., "The Presidential Address—Chaplaincy in Transition: The Second 25 Years," *Bulletin of the American Protestant Hospital Association,* Vol. XXXVI, No. 2 (1972), p. 2.

4. Robert A. Lambourne, "With Love to the U.S.A.," *Journal of Religion and Health,* Vol. VIII, No. 4 (Oct. 1969).

5. *Ibid.,* p. 316.

6. Seward Hiltner, "An Appraisal of the Lambourne Appraisal," *Journal of Religion and Health,* Vol. VIII, No. 4 (Oct. 1969), p. 330.

7. George W. Webber, "On the Way to Tomorrow," *Bulletin of the American Protestant Hospital Association,* Vol. XXXVII, No. 2 (1973), p. 18.

8. Carroll A. Wise, "The Chaplain of the Future," in Holst and Kurtz, *op. cit.,* p. 140.

9. See Lambourne, *op. cit.,* pp. 313f.

10. Roy Branson, "Bioethics as Individual and Social: The Scope of a Consulting Profession and Academic Discipline," *The Journal of Religious Ethics,* Vol. III, No. 1 (1975), p. 122. Branson traces the interesting and significant parallels of biomedical ethics with the disciplines of the history of medicine and the sociology of medicine.

11. I am indebted to the suggestive treatment of some of these theological themes by Robert V. Moss, "The Role of the Church in the Health Care System," address given to the National Association of Health and Welfare Ministries, March 1975 (mimeographed).

12. *Ibid.,* p. 3.

13. *Ibid.*

14. Heije Faber, *Pastoral Care in the Modern Hospital* (Philadelphia: The Westminster Press, 1971), pp. 81ff.

15. See Thomas A. Harris, "The Chaplain: Prophet, Jester, or Jerk," *Bulletin of the American Protestant Hospital Association,* Vol. XXXVI, No. 2 (1972).

16. *Ibid.,* p. 48.

CHAPTER 4: Personal Needs of Patients

1. I have dealt with these concerns in more detail in *Human Medicine* (Minneapolis: Augsburg Publishing House, 1973), pp. 13ff.

2. A hopeful sign that fresh consideration is beginning to occur is found in the essays in John Y. Fenton (ed.), *Theology and Body* (Philadelphia: The Westminster Press, 1974). See esp. Sam Keen's remarks, pp. 18f.

3. See Robert V. Moss, "The Role of the Church in the Health Care System," address given to the National Association of Health and Welfare Ministries, March 1975 (mimeographed), pp. 4f.

4. For a fuller treatment of the notion of caring, see Milton Mayeroff, *On Caring* (New York: Harper & Row, 1971). Cf. my *Human Medicine,* pp. 28ff.

5. See Erik H. Erikson, *Childhood and Society* (2nd Edition) (New York: W. W. Norton and Company, Inc., 1963), pp. 247-274; and Richard I. Evans, *Dialogue with Erik Erikson* (New York: Harper & Row, 1967), pp. 11-58.

6. This case is described by Robert Belknap, the physician in the situation, in "A Dying Patient," *Synthesis,* Vol. I, No. 1 (1975), pp. 82ff. The applications of Erikson's categories are mine.

7. Erikson, *Childhood and Society,* p. 269.

8. Lois Jaffe, herself a leukemia victim, has discussed these and numerous related issues in a remarkable essay, "Sexual Problems of the Terminally Ill," soon to be published.

9. JoAnn Kelley Smith, *Free Fall* (Valley Forge, Pennsylvania: Judson Press, 1975), p. 106.

10. David Cole Gordon, *Self-Love* (Baltimore: Penguin Books, Inc., 1968, 1972), p. 9.

CHAPTER 5: Bodies, Sexuality, and Personal Health

1. World Health Organization, *Education and Treatment in Human Sexuality: The Training of Health Professionals* (Geneva: World Health Organization, 1975), p. 6.

2. *Ibid.*

3. Daniel H. Labby, M.D., "Sexual Concomitants of Disease and Illness," *Postgraduate Medicine,* Vol. 58, No. 1 (July 1975), p. 103.

4. Richard A. Chilgren, M.D., "Sexuality and Beyond," *ibid.,* p. 46. This symposium issue of *Postgraduate Medicine* on "Sexuality and Sexual Health," guest-edited by Chilgren and James W. Maddock, Ph.D., is a valuable resource for medical insights on this subject.

5. D. H. Lawrence, *Lady Chatterley's Lover* (New York: Pocket Books, Inc., 1959), p. 83. Cf. Leslie Paul's comments on this passage in his *Eros Rediscovered: Restoring Sex to Humanity* (New York: Association Press, 1970), p. 131.

6. See Hans Hofmann, *Sex Incorporated* (Boston: Beacon Press, 1967), pp. 3ff. for a further elaboration of this distinction.

7. Harvey Gallagher Cox, Jr., "Sexuality and Responsibility: A New Phase," in John Charles Wynn (ed.) *Sexual Ethics and Christian Responsibility* (New York: Association Press, 1970), Chap. 2.

8. Rollo May, *Love and Will* (New York: W. W. Norton & Co., Inc., 1969), Chaps. 1 and 2.

9. James W. Maddock, Ph.D., "Sexual Health and Health Care," *Postgraduate Medicine, op. cit.,* p. 53.

10. Quoted by Rollo May, *Paulus: Reminiscences of a Friendship* (New York: Harper & Row, Publishers, 1973), p. 38.

11. Michael Novak, *Ascent of the Mountain, Flight of the Dove* (New York: Harper & Row, Publishers, 1971), p. 25. Cf. Eric Mount, Jr., *The Feminine Factor* (Richmond, Virginia: John Knox Press, 1973), pp. 138f.

12. H. Richard Niebuhr raised this question. See his *Radical Monotheism and Western Culture* (New York: Harper and Brothers, Publishers, 1960).

13. Rosemary Reuther, "An Unexpected Tribute to the Theologian," *Theology Today,* Vol. 27, No. 3 (October 1970), pp. 337ff., as cited in Mount, pp. 137f.

14. See Mount, p. 138. Mount's fine book draws together a wide range of sources on this issue. See also John Y. Fenton, *Theology and Body* (Philadelphia: The Westminster Press, 1974).

15. Quoted in Paul, pp. 148f.

16. See Lawrence Merideth, *The Sensuous Christian* (New York: Association Press, 1972), p. 105.

17. See Abel Jeanniere, *The Anthropology of Sex,* trans. Julie Kernan (New York: Harper & Row, Publishers, 1967), pp. 15f.

18. Cf. Paul, pp. 142f.

19. Jeanniere, p. 15.

20. Tom F. Driver, "Sexuality and Jesus," in Martin E. Marty and Dean G. Peerman (eds.), *New Theology No. 3* (New York: The Macmillan Company, 1966); also "On Taking Sex Seriously," *Christianity and Crisis,* Vol. 23 (October 14, 1963).

21. Dan Sullivan, Introduction to Jeanniere, *The Anthropology of Sex,* p. 17.

22. John A. T. Robinson, *The Human Face of God* (Philadelphia: The Westminster Press, 1973), p. 64.

23. Robinson urges that a reassessment of the Virgin Birth mythos is important in this regard. If we interpret the Virgin Birth as a non-literal way of attempting to affirm something about Jesus as the Christ, we are left, according to Robinson, with only three possibilities concerning Jesus' conception. One is that Joseph was his human father who impregnated Mary inside wedlock; another is that Joseph impregnated Mary outside wedlock and subsequently legitimized this action by marriage. But both of these possibilities are not strongly supported by biblical evidence. Hence, a third possibility presents itself: that the conception took place outside wedlock by an unknown party, and this was subsequently accepted by Joseph. In pressing this point, Robinson may be stretching the evidence too far. Nevertheless, his overall contention concerning the radical scandal of the Incarnation is clear and appropriate. See *Ibid.,* pp. 57ff.

24. See *Ibid.,* pp. 197ff.

25. *Ibid.,* p. 199.

26. *Ibid.,* p. 16.

27. Rosemary Reuther, "Mother Earth and the Megamachine," *Christianity and Crisis,* Vol. 31, No. 21 (December 13, 1971), p. 269. Cf. Mount, p. 112.

28. Mount provides a most helpful detailing of some of these implications. See his Chaps. 3 and 4.

29. Paul Tillich, *The Shaking of the Foundations* (New York: Charles Scribner's Sons, 1948), p. 162.

30. Driver, "Sexuality and Jesus," p. 125. Driver's insights on the nature of Jesus' love are extremely helpful.

31. Abraham Maslow, "Love in Self-Actualizing People," in Hendrik M. Ruitenbeek (ed.), *Sexuality and Identity* (New York: Dell Publishing Co., Inc., 1970). This quotation and those which follow are found on pp. 224-233.

32. From *Our Town* by Thornton Wilder. Copyright 1938, 1957 by Thornton Wilder. By permission of Harper and Row.

CHAPTER 6: Personhood, Decisions, and Death

1. For a fuller discussion of this issue, see my *Human Medicine* (Minneapolis: Augsburg Publishing House, 1973), pp. 130ff.

2. *Minutes of the General Synod,* United Church of Christ, St. Louis, Missouri, June 22-26, 1973, p. 42.

3. See Daniel C. Maguire, *Death by Choice* (Garden City, N.Y.: Doubleday & Co., Inc., 1974), Chap. 5; and Paul Ramsey, *The Patient as Person* (New Haven: Yale University Press, 1970), Chap. 3; both of these ethicists make arguments in favor of maintaining the omission/commission distinction. Joseph Fletcher, on the other hand, has long argued that the distinction is not ethically significant because of the agent's intentionality: *Morals and Medicine* (Boston: Beacon Press, 1960), Chap. 6; and *Moral Responsibility* (Philadelphia: The Westminster Press, 1967), Chap. IX. Cf. philosopher James Rachel's similar argument in "Active and Passive Euthanasia," *The New England Journal of Medicine,* Vol. 292, No. 2 (Jan. 9, 1975), pp. 78ff. It is interesting to note that while most physicians who associate *commission* with *withdrawal* of medical supports disapprove of withdrawal on those grounds, not all do. An exception is illustrated in these lines written by Thomas W. Furlow, Jr., M.D., University of Virginia, who elsewhere argues for the acceptance of active euthanasia: "For example, if a physician discontinues a vital treatment

in progress on a dying but vegetatively alive patient (e.g. 'pulling the plug'), that physician is said to have performed passive euthanasia. Yet, by commission of his act, I contend that this physician has carried out active euthanasia just as surely as if he had given the patient a dose of potassium cyanide." "Correspondence," *The New England Journal of Medicine,* Vol. 292, No. 16 (April 17, 1975), p. 866.

4. Ramsey, *op. cit.,* p. 121.

5. For fuller discussions, see *Human Medicine,* pp. 131f., Ramsey, *op. cit.,* pp. 118ff., and Gerald Kelly, S.J., *Medico-Moral Problems* (St. Louis: The Catholic Hospital Association, 1958), p. 129.

6. It is worth noting that some ethicists prefer to keep the lines between ordinary and heroic more tightly drawn. Instead of saying that in some situations the nature of the progressing illness can cause what was once ordinary to be considered now heroic, they say that the situation of the particular illness may dictate that even ordinary measures become out of place, useless, or positively harmful to personhood. Either way, the ethical result is the same. Cf. Gerald Kelly, S.J., "The Duty of Using Artificial Means of Preserving Life," *Theological Studies,* Vol. 11 (June 1950). Some physicians and ethicists, however, argue that the terms "reasonable" and "unreasonable" are more appropriate than ordinary and extraordinary. Willard Gaylin, for example, says, "Reasonable has meaning only within the matrix of the individual, the quality of the life that will be sustained and the values of both the individual and the society that define that quality." Whichever terms are used, the important point is that they refer to appropriateness or inappropriateness *for a particular patient.* The terms ought never be interpreted as referring to technological devices as such. Willard Gaylin, et al, "The Case of Karen Quinlan," *Christianity and Crisis,* Vol. 35, No. 22 (Jan. 19, 1976), pp. 324, 329.

7. Daniel C. Maguire gives an excellent and more extended discussion of these persons and groups in Chap. 8, *op. cit.* I am dependent on him for some of the ideas expressed here.

8. See Howard Brody, *Ethical Decisions in Medicine* (Boston: Little, Brown and Company, 1976), p. 204.

9. William A. Nolen, M.D., "What Your Doctor Owes You," *Mc-Calls,* Vol. 102. No. 10 (July 1975), p. 17.

10. *Op. cit.,* p. 179. Maguire discusses more fully some of the ideas expressed in the following paragraph.

11. See *ibid.,* p. 181.

12. Cited in *ibid.*

13. See *ibid.,* pp. 184f.

14. See the summaries of the state of the law and legal practice in Jerry B. Wilson, *Death by Decision: The Medical, Moral, and Legal Dilemmas of Euthanasia* (Philadelphia: The Westminster Press, 1975), pp. 149ff; Marya Mannes, *Last Rights: A Case for the Good Death* (New York: New American Library, 1973), pp. 116ff; and in Maguire, *op. cit.,* pp. 45ff.

15. For insightful commentary on the lower court's decision by several physicians and ethicists, see *The Hastings Center Report,* Vol. 6, No. 1 (February 1976).

16. *In the Matter of Karen Quinlan, An Alleged Incompetent,* A-116, Supreme Court of New Jersey (March 31, 1976), p. 37.

17. *Ibid.,* p. 42.

18. *Ibid.,* p. 47.

19. *Ibid.,* p. 48.

20. *Ibid.,* pp. 53f.

21. *Ibid.,* pp. 57f. In spite of the remarkable clarity of most of the second Quinlan decision, some confusion unfortunately remains over the composition and functioning of the "Ethics Committee." Regarding its composition, at one point (p. 50) the court appears to suggest that it be interdisciplinary, including physicians, social workers, attorneys, and theologians. Elsewhere, however (p. 51), the court compares the committee to "multi-judge courts," which are obviously not interdisciplinary in their composition. The issue is significant. If, on the one hand, such a committee is to function as an *ethics* committee with value decisions as a major concern, it clearly ought to be interdisciplinary in its makeup. On the other hand, in this particular case the court actually charged such

a committee with the task of verifying the *medical* prognosis of the patient, a matter which is not essentially a value decision nor one appropriate to non-physicians. Second, the court says, "although the deliberations and decisions which we describe would be professional in nature they should obviously include at some stage the feelings of the family of an incompetent relative" (p. 52). This wording can be construed to mean that it is finally the committee which makes the decision whether or not to remove the extraordinary medical supports. However, in making Joseph Quinlan the guardian of the person of his daughter, the court also made it clear that he had "full power to make decisions with regard to the identity of her treating physicians" (p. 58). This certainly appears to mean that the final decisional power is lodged with the family, for they would be free to change physicians and even to move their daughter to a different hospital and hence to deal with a different ethics committee. Because the nature and functioning of such ethics committees is of great importance for similar future cases, and because it is crucial that no doubt be left about the *prima facie* rights of the family in such situations, this matter deserves further clarification. As we have seen, families *can* make decisions which are not in the best interests of the patient. In such instances, as in the Jehovah's Witnesses blood transfusion cases, the state can rightly intervene. But in a free and pluralistic society where the integrity of the family unit should be honored, we should assume that families do act in the best interests of their members until proven otherwise.

22. *Ibid.*, p. 52.

CHAPTER 7: Persons, Values, and Medicine

1. *Time,* Vol. 105, No. 25 (June 16, 1975), p. 49.

2. As quoted in *The Los Angeles Times,* April 9, 1975, p. 3.

3. Irvine H. Page, M.D., "Ethical Troubles: Who's Making the Rules?" *Modern Medicine,* Vol. 42, No. 8 (April 15, 1974), p. 33.

4. William A. Nolen, M.D., "What Your Doctor Owes You," *McCalls,* Vol. 102, No. 10 (July 1975), p. 17.

5. Niebuhr's writings on love and justice are found in numerous of

his books and articles. One of his particularly fine statements is found in *The Nature and Destiny of Man: Vol. II, Human Destiny* (New York: Charles Scribner's Sons, 1943), Chap. IX.

6. *Time, op. cit.,* p. 50.

7. John G. Bruhn and Douglas C. Smith, "Social Ethics for Medical Educators," in Maurice B. Visscher (ed.), *Humanistic Perspectives in Medical Ethics* (Buffalo: Prometheus Books, 1972), p. 293.

8. Daniel Callahan, "The WHO Definition of Health," *Hastings Center Studies* Vol. 1, No. 3 (1973), esp. p. 83.

9. Robert M. Veatch, "The Medical Model: Its Nature and Problems," *Hastings Center Studies,* Vol. 1, No. 3 (1973), p. 73. See also Paul Ramsey, *The Patient as Person* (New Haven: Yale University Press, 1970), pp. 123f.

10. See Peter Sedgwick, "Medical Individualism," *Hastings Center Studies,* Vol. 2, No. 3 (1974), p. 73. This entire issue on "The Future of Individualism" is a valuable resource on this matter.

11. Victor W. Sidel and Ruth Sidel, "Medicine in China: Individual and Society," *Hastings Center Studies,* Vol. 2, No. 3 (1974), p. 23.

12. *Ibid.,* p. 35.

13. These goals are those of the Lutheran Council in the U.S.A. Their statement on national health care policy is an excellent example of church statements on this issue. See *Health Care for All Americans! Testimony given by the Lutheran Council in the U.S.A. to the Committee on Ways and Means, U. S. House of Representatives,* July 2, 1974.

14. See, for example, Henry Miller, *Medicine and Society* (London: Oxford University Press, 1973), Chap. 4; see also the monthly publication *Contact* of the Christian Medical Commission, World Council of Churches.

15. Walter Brueggemann, "Healing and Caring," *Engage/Social Action,* Vol. 2, No. 7 (July 1974), pp. 14-24. Prof. Brueggemann's insightful biblical interpretation has guided my thinking in these three paragraphs.